Fariza Halimova
Firuz Shukurov

Course of lectures on normal physiology. Volume two

Fariza Halimova
Firuz Shukurov

Course of lectures on normal physiology. Volume two

ScienciaScripts

Imprint
Any brand names and product names mentioned in this book are subject to trademark, brand or patent protection and are trademarks or registered trademarks of their respective holders. The use of brand names, product names, common names, trade names, product descriptions etc. even without a particular marking in this work is in no way to be construed to mean that such names may be regarded as unrestricted in respect of trademark and brand protection legislation and could thus be used by anyone.

Cover image: www.ingimage.com

This book is a translation from the original published under ISBN 978-620-7-64141-3.

Publisher:
Sciencia Scripts
is a trademark of
Dodo Books Indian Ocean Ltd. and OmniScriptum S.R.L publishing group

120 High Road, East Finchley, London, N2 9ED, United Kingdom
Str. Armeneasca 28/1, office 1, Chisinau MD-2012, Republic of Moldova, Europe
Printed at: see last page
ISBN: 978-620-7-62289-4

KHALIMOVA FARIZA TURSUNBAEVNA
SHUKUROV FIRUZ ABDUFATTOEVICH,

LECTURE COURSE ON NORMAL PHYSIOLOGY

Volume Two

Table of Contents

Lectures, this is a continuation of the published lectures on normal physiology in 2023 by Lambert Publishers. The lectures are numbered from the first volume of the lectures.

Lecture 21.

Topic: Motor and absorptive function of the GI tract.

Objective - to know the types of movement of the different parts of the digestive tract and the physiologic mechanisms of absorption

Objectives - (a) To disclose the types of movement of different parts of the digestive tract, their role in digestion;

b) show the mechanisms of absorption;

c) review the characteristics of fat absorption

Content:

Chewing is the process of mechanical processing of food between the upper and lower rows of teeth through the movement of the lower jaw relative to the upper jaw. Chewing is accomplished by contraction of masticatory and mimic muscles, as well as muscles of the tongue. Impulses from the receptors of the oral cavity come through the sensitive fibers of the trigeminal nerve to the center of mastication, which is located in the medulla oblongata. Impulses from here on the motor fibers of the trigeminal nerve come to the masticatory muscles - they carry out the movement of the lower jaw. The muscles of the tongue, cheeks and lips move the food ball in the mouth, feed and hold food between the chewing surfaces of the teeth. The substantia nigra and the cerebral cortex play a major role in coordinating the act of chewing.

At registration of mastication the following phases are revealed: resting, introduction of food into the mouth, tentative, basic, formation of a food clump. Each phase and the whole period of chewing have different duration and character, which depends on the properties and amount of chewed food, age, appetite, individual characteristics, fullness of the chewing apparatus and mechanisms of its control.

Swallowing is the passage of a food clump from the mouth to the stomach. When the receptors of the oral cavity are irritated, the sensory fibers of the trigeminal, laryngeal and lingual nerves impulses arrive in the medulla oblongata, where the swallowing center is located. From here, impulses on efferent fibers of the trigeminal, lingual, hyoid and vagus nerves reach the muscles that provide the act of swallowing. Bulbar center is coordinated by the motor centers of the midbrain and cerebral cortex. The swallowing center is in close communication with the respiratory center, inhibiting it during swallowing, which prevents food from entering the airways. The swallowing reflex consists of three phases:

Mouth (arbitrary) - in this phase the formation of a food clump with a volume of 5 - 15 cm takes place. By movement of the tongue it is moved to its back. By arbitrary contractions of the front and then middle part of the tongue, the food ball is pressed against the hard palate and transferred to the root of the tongue.

Pharyngeal (fast, short involuntary) in this case, irritation of the root of the tongue reflexively causes contraction of the muscles that raise the soft palate, which prevents food from entering the nasal cavity. Movements of the tongue food lump is pushed into the pharynx. At the same time there is a contraction of the muscles that dislocate the hyoid bone and cause the larynx to rise, which closes the entrance to the airways, which prevents the entry of food into them. Following the entry of the food clump into the pharynx, there is a contraction of the muscles that narrow its lumen above the food clump, as a result of which it moves into the esophagus. Before swallowing the pharyngeal-esophageal sphincter is closed, during swallowing the pressure in the pharynx rises to 45 mm Hg, the sphincter opens and the food lump enters the beginning of the esophagus, where the pressure is no more than 30 mm Hg. These two phases of swallowing last 1s.

Esophageal (slow, prolonged involuntary) - during this phase the food clump moves down the esophagus and is transferred to the stomach. Duration of this phase 8 - 9s (liquid food 1 - 2s). Outside of swallowing, the entrance from the esophagus to the stomach is closed by the lower esophageal sphincter. The movements of the esophagus are caused reflexively with each swallowing act. The contractions of the esophagus have a wave character, originating in its upper part and spreading towards the stomach. This type of contraction is called peristaltic. This type of contraction occurs due to the coordinated contraction of the annular (circular) muscles of the esophagus (above the food clump) and longitudinal (below the food clump). Parasympathetic fibers of the vagus nerve stimulate esophageal peristalsis and relax the cardiac portion of the stomach. Sympathetic fibers inhibit esophageal motility and increase cardiac tone.

Gastric motor function.

During and in the first few minutes after a meal, the stomach relaxes, allowing food to be deposited. The stomach has two pacemakers that regulate motor function: the *cardiac* pacemaker and the *pyloric* pacemaker. Three types of movements occur in a filled stomach:

Peristaltic waves, their frequency is 3 in 1 min, they propagate from the cardiac part to the pyloric part at a speed of 1 cm/s. During the first hour after ingestion these waves are weak, later they intensify. At the same time, the pressure in the pyloric section increases to 10 - 25 cm of water column, the sphincter opens and a portion of chyme leaves the stomach into the 12-peristal colon. The remaining amount of chyme returns to the proximal pyloric portion of the stomach. This type of movement provides mixing and grinding of food contents, provides homogenization of chyme.

Systolic contractions of the pyloric section (pyloric or staminal reflex). When the stomach is empty, the pyloric sphincter is in a relaxed state. After the transition of the first portion of chyme from the stomach to the 12-peristaltic colon due to peristaltic waves, there is a reflex contraction of the sphincter (pyloric reflex) and stops the exit of chyme from the stomach. The main stimulus of the pyloric reflex is hydrochloric acid, which together with chyme enters the 12-pearl intestine. Impulses from chemoreceptors go to the medulla oblongata and the efferent impulsation along the vagus nerve to the pyloric sphincter increases. It should be noted that the rate of evacuation of chyme from the stomach into the 12-intestine depends on many factors: volume, composition, consistency, the value of osmotic pressure, temperature and pH content, the pressure gradient between the cavities of the stomach and 12-intestine. Food rich in carbohydrates is evacuated faster from the stomach than rich in proteins. Fatty foods are evacuated at the lowest rate. The time of complete evacuation of mixed food is 6 to 10 hours.

Tonic contractions to help reduce the cavity of the fundus and body of the stomach.

The regulation of gastric motility is accomplished by two main mechanisms:

1) *nerve regulation* - accomplished by the vagus nerve (increases gastric motility) and sympathetic nerve (inhibits gastric motility);

2) *humoral regulation* - gastric motility is enhanced by gastrin, motilin, serotonin, insulin, and inhibited by secretin, glucagon, and VIP. The mechanism of their influence is direct (direct influence on muscle bundles) and indirect - through intramural neurons.

Vomiting is the involuntary release of the contents of the digestive tract through the mouth (sometimes the nose as well). Vomiting occurs in two phases: *1st phase is intestinal.* It involves antiperistaltic contractions of the small intestine and the intestinal contents are pushed into the stomach (reflux). After 10 to 20 seconds, the *2nd phase (gastric phase)* begins. In this case there is a contraction of the stomach, opens the cardiac section, after a deep inhalation strongly contract the muscles of the abdominal wall and diaphragm and the contents of the stomach at the time of exhalation ejected through the esophagus into the mouth. Vomiting has a protective value and occurs reflexively when irritated by the root of the tongue, pharynx, gastric mucosa, biliary tract, peritoneum, coronary vessels, vestibular apparatus. It may arise from the action of certain substances on the nerve center of vomiting. The vomiting center is located at the bottom of the IV ventricle in the reticular formation of the medulla oblongata. Efferent impulses that provide vomiting, follow to the intestine, stomach and esophagus as part of the vagus and phrenic nerves, as well as nerves innervating the abdominal and diaphragmatic muscles, muscles of the trunk and limbs, which provides basic and auxiliary movements, including the characteristic posture.

Motor function of the small intestine. This function provides chyme pulverization, mixing of chyme with intestinal juice, chyme advancement, and increased intraintestinal pressure that promotes filtration of solutes from the intestinal cavity into the blood and lymph. Thus the motility of the small intestine contributes to the hydrolysis and absorption of nutrients. The following types of movement are distinguished:

Rhythmic segmentation - this movement is carried out due to the predominant contraction of the circular layer of muscles (p.32, FigZh2A). In this case, a small segment of the intestine is divided into many segments of 1.5 - 2 cm each. This type of movement ensures that the chyme is pulverized.

Pendulum-like movement - is carried out mainly due to the contraction of longitudinal muscles (p.32, Fig.Zh2B). Due to this movement the mixing of chyme with intestinal juice takes place.

Peristaltic movement - is carried out by coordinated contraction of circular and longitudinal muscles. Due to this movement, chyme moves through the intestine.

Tonic contractions - may be localized or may move at a very low speed. Tonic contractions narrow the intestinal lumen over a large length of the intestine (this type of contraction differs from rhythmic segmentation) and contributes to increased pressure in the intestine.

Antiperistaltic contractions - in this case, the peristaltic wave moves in the opposite (oral) direction. Normally, this type of contraction does not occur. This type of contraction is characteristic of vomiting.

The regulation of intestinal motility is realized by the following mechanisms: myogenic, nervous and humoral. The *myogenic mechanism is* provided due to the automaticity of intestinal smooth muscles, which begin to contract when the intestine is distended. The phasic contractile activity of the intestinal wall is provided by neurons of the muscular-intestinal (auerbachian) nerve plexus, which have rhythmic background activity. It should be noted that in addition to this metasympathetic plexus there are two more "sensors" of the rhythm of intestinal contractions: at the place of the common bile duct flowing into the 12-peristal colon and in the ileum. *Nervous regulation is* carried out by parasympathetic nerves (mainly increase intestinal motility) and sympathetic nerves (inhibit intestinal motility).

Humoral regulation is accomplished by serotonin, histamine, gastrin, motilin, vasopressin, oxytacin, bradykinin (increase intestinal motility), secretin, and VMP (inhibit intestinal motility).

In addition to the above mechanisms in the regulation of small intestinal motility play a role:

1) *local stimuli in the* form of products of digestion of nutrients (fats, acids, alkalis, salts), which increase intestinal motility;

2) *reflexes* from different parts of the digestive tract: esophageal-intestinal (enhances), gastrointestinal (enhances and inhibits), recto-enteral (inhibits);

3) the *act of eating* - first inhibits and then increases intestinal motility. Further it is determined by the physical and chemical properties of chyme: coarse, rich in undigested in the small intestine dietary fibers and fats food increases intestinal motility.

Motor function of the large intestine. The entire process of digestion in an adult lasts 1 - 3 days, of which the most time is spent on the stay of food residues in the large intestine. Motility of the large intestine provides reservoir function (accumulation of contents), absorption of a number of substances from it (mainly water), its promotion, the formation of feces and their removal (defecation). The large intestine fills up within 24 h and empties completely in 48 - 72 h.

In the colon, the following types of contractions are distinguished: *small and large pendulum-like, peristaltic, propulsive and antiperistaltic.* These movements (except antiperistaltic) provide mixing of the intestinal contents and increase the pressure in its cavity. This promotes thickening of the contents by absorption of water. Strong *propulsive* contractions occur 3 to 4 times a day and propel the intestinal contents distally.

Parasympathetic innervation (as part of the vagus and pelvic nerves) enhances motility through conditioned and unconditional reflexes when the esophagus, stomach and small intestine are irritated. Sympathetic nerves (as part of the phrenic nerves) inhibit motility of the intestine.

Defecation is the emptying of feces from the large intestine, resulting from the irritation of the receptors of the rectum by the accumulated feces in it. The urge to defecate occurs when the pressure in the rectum increases to 40 - 50 cm of water. A pressure of 20 to 30 cm of water causes a feeling of filling of the rectum. There are two sphincters in the rectum: *internal*, consisting of smooth muscles, and *external*, formed by transverse striated muscles. Outside the act of defecation, these sphincters are in a state of tonic contraction. The act of defecation occurs due to relaxation of these sphincters, peristaltic contractions of the intestine, contraction of the muscle that raises the anus (there is a shortening of the distal part of the rectum) and contraction of its ring muscles. In the act of defecation is of great importance *pushing*, which contract the muscles of the abdominal wall and diaphragm, increasing intra-abdominal pressure, reaching up to 220 cm of water. The primary reflex arc closes in the lumbosacral spinal cord and provides an involuntary act of defecation. The arbitrary act is carried out with the participation of the cortex of the large hemispheres, centers of the medulla oblongata and hypothalamus. Parasympathetic nerves (as part of the pelvic nerve) inhibits sphincter tone and increases rectal motility, stimulating the act of defecation. Sympathetic nerves increase sphincter tone and inhibit rectal motility. The arbitrary component of the act of defecation consists of downward influences of the brain on the spinal center, resulting in relaxation of the external sphincter, contraction of the diaphragm and abdominal muscles. In healthy people, the act of defecation is performed 1 to 2 times a day.

Colonic gas. In a day from the intestine during defecation and outside of it is removed 100 - 500 ml of gas. With flatulence, its volume can reach 3 liters and more. Stretching of the large intestine gas causes a state of discomfort, a feeling of bloating. Stretching the small intestine with gas causes pain. A significant amount of gas is formed in the intestine. When the hydrocarbonates of the pancreatic secretion interact with acidic products of intestinal chyme, a significant amount of CO is formed$_2$. Gases are also produced by the intestinal microflora. During digestion of some types of food (beans, cabbage, black bread, potatoes) with the participation of microflora a large amount of gases is formed. In healthy people, the gas mixture leaving the intestine includes: N_2 (24 - 90%), CO_2 (4 - 29%), O_2 (up to 23%), H_2 (0.6 - 47%), methane (0 - 26%), a small amount of hydrogen sulfide, ammonia, mercaptan.

Absorption is a set of processes that ensure the transfer of various substances into the blood and lymph from the digestive tract. Absorbed substances are spread throughout the body and are included in the metabolism of tissues. Absorption of different substances are carried out by different mechanisms. Absorption of macromolecules and their aggregates occurs by *phagocytosis and pinocytosis.* These mechanisms are related to *endocytosis.* Intracellular digestion is associated with endocytosis. A number of substances, having entered the cell by endocytosis, are transported in a vesicle through the cell and released from it by *exocytosis* into the intercellular space. Such transport of substances is called *transcytosis.* This transport is not essential in nutrient transport. However, immunoglobulins, vitamins, and enzymes are transported from the intestine into the blood by this mechanism. In newborns, transcytosis is important in the transport of breast milk proteins. Some substances can be transported through intercellular spaces - such transport is called *persorption.* Some water, electrolytes, some proteins (antibodies, allergens, enzymes) and bacteria are transported by persorption. Micromolecules are mainly transported from the gastrointestinal tract: nutrient monomers and ions. This transport is carried out by the following mechanisms: *active transport; passive transport; facilitated diffusion.*

Active transport is the transfer of substances across membranes against concentration, osmotic and electrochemical gradients with the expenditure of energy and with the participation of special transport systems: mobile transporters, conformational transporters and membrane transport channels. Membranes have transporters of many types. Sodium ions are most often used in such a role. Sodium dependent process in the small intestine is the absorption of glucose, galactose, free amino acids, dipeptides, tripeptides, bile acid salts, and bilirubin. Sodium dependent transport is accomplished through specialized channels and by mobile transporters. Sodium-dependent transporters are located on apical membranes, and sodium pumps are located on basolateral membranes of enterocytes

Passive transport is carried out without energy input by concentration, osmotic and electrochemical gradients and includes: *diffusion, filtration, osmosis. The* driving force of *diffusion of* dissolved matter particles is their concentration gradient. A type of diffusion is *osmosis, in* which the movement occurs in accordance with the concentration gradient of solvent particles. *Filtration is* understood as the process of solute transport through a porous membrane under the action of hydrostatic pressure.

Facilitated diffusion, as well as simple diffusion, is carried out without energy expenditure along the concentration gradient. However, facilitated diffusion is a faster process and is carried out with the participation of special membrane transporters.

The rate of absorption depends on the properties of the intestinal contents: absorption is faster when the intestinal contents are neutral than when they are acidic or alkaline; absorption of electrolytes and nutrients is faster from an isotonic environment than from hypo- and hypertonic environments.

An increase in intraintestinal pressure increases the rate of absorption of table salt solution from the small intestine. This indicates the importance of filtration in absorption and intestinal motility.

Absorption in different parts of the digestive tract

In the oral cavity, absorption is practically absent due to the short stay of substances in it and the absence of monomeric hydrolysis products. The oral mucosa is permeable to sodium, potassium, some amino acids, alcohol, some drugs.

In the stomach, the intensity of absorption is also low. Water and dissolved mineral salts are absorbed here. In addition, weak solutions of alcohol and some medicines are absorbed in the stomach.

In the duodenum, the intensity of absorption is greater than in the stomach, but not by much.

The main process of absorption (nutrients, water, electrolytes) occurs in the jejunum and ileum. In the mechanism of absorption in the small intestine, the contraction of villi of the small intestinal mucosa and microvilli of enterocytes are of special importance. By contractions of villi, lymph with substances absorbed into it is squeezed out of the shrinking cavity of lymphatic vessels. The presence of valves in them prevents the return of lymph into the vessel at the subsequent relaxation of villi and creates a suction action of the central lymphatic vessel. Contraction of the microvilli enhances endocytosis. On an empty stomach, villi contract rarely and weakly. In the presence of chyme in the intestine, the contraction of villi is intensified and more frequent. Mechanical irritation of the base of villi and under the influence of chemical components of food, especially products of its hydrolysis (peptides, some amino acids, glucose and extractive substances of food) and bile acids influence the strength of villi contraction. The intramural nervous system (submucosal or Meissner plexus) plays a role in enhancing villus contraction. The main humoral factor that stimulates the contraction of villi is the hormone *vilikinin,* which is formed in the mucosa of the 12-intestine under the influence of acidic gastric contents on the small intestine. Absorption depends on the size of the surface on which it takes place. In humans, the surface of the mucosa of the small intestine is increased 300-500 times due to folds, villi and microvilli. There are 30-40 villi per 1 mm^2 of intestinal mucosa, and each enterocyte has 1700-4000 microvilli. There are 50-100 million microvilli per 1 mm^2 surface of the intestinal epithelium.

Absorption of various substances in the small intestine:

Absorption of water and mineral salts. Water enters the digestive tract as part of food and drinking liquids (2 - 2.5 liters), digestive gland secretions (6 - 7 liters), is eliminated with feces 100 - 150 ml. The rest of the water is absorbed from the digestive tract into the blood, a small amount in the lymph. Absorption of water begins in the stomach, but more intensively in the small intestine and especially in the large intestine (per day about 8 liters). The decisive role in water transport belongs to the sodium ion. The sodium pump inhibitor ouabain inhibits water absorption. Water absorption is also associated with the transport of sugars and amino acids. For example, suppression of sugars absorption by floricin slows water absorption. Dietary intake of water is altered. Increasing the proportion of protein in it increases the rate of absorption of water, sodium and chlorine.

More than 1 mole of sodium chloride is absorbed in the gastrointestinal tract per day. In humans, sodium is almost not absorbed in the stomach, intensively absorbed in the large intestine and ileum, in the jejunum its absorption is much less. Sodium enters the blood from the cavity of the small intestine both through intestinal epitheliocytes and through intercellular channels. In the large intestine, sodium absorption is independent of the content of sugars and amino acids, but in the small intestine it is.

Potassium absorption occurs mainly in the small intestine by means of active and passive transport mechanisms along the electrochemical gradient. Absorption of chlorine ions occurs in the stomach and most actively in the ileum by active and passive transport. Passive transport is conjugated with the transport of sodium ions. Active transport is carried out through the apical membranes and is associated with the transport of sodium ions or the exchange of chlorine ions for the NCO ion$_3$. Divalent ions are absorbed very slowly in the digestive tract.

Absorption of protein hydrolysis products. Proteins are mainly absorbed in the intestine after their hydrolysis to amino acids. Absorption of different amino acids occurs at different rates in different parts of the small intestine. The fastest absorbed are arginine, methionine, leucine, slower - phenylalanine, cysteine, tyrosine, even slower - alanine, serine, glutamic acid. L-forms of amino acids are absorbed more intensively than D-forms. Absorption of amino acids from the intestine into epithelial cells through apical membranes is carried out actively with the help of transporters with considerable energy expenditure of phosphorus-containing macroergens. A small fraction of amino acids are absorbed passively by diffusion. Several types of amino acid transporters exist in the apical membranes of epitheliocytes. From epitheliocytes, amino acids are transported into the intercellular fluid by a facilitated diffusion mechanism. Amino acids formed during hydrolysis of proteins and peptides are absorbed more rapidly than free amino acids introduced into the small intestine. Sodium transport stimulates the absorption of amino acids. Amino acids absorbed into the bloodstream travel through the portal vein system to the liver, where they undergo various transformations. A significant portion of amino acids is used for protein synthesis. Amino acids in the liver are deaminated, and some undergo enzymatic overamination. Amino acids are distributed throughout the body and serve as starting material for the construction of various tissue proteins, hormones, enzymes, hemoglobin and other substances of protein nature. Some amino acids are used as a source of energy.

The intensity of amino acid absorption depends on age (more intensively at a young age), the level of protein metabolism in the body, the content of free amino acids in the blood from nervous and humoral influences.

Absorption of carbohydrates. Glucose and galactose (hexoses) are absorbed at the highest rate, while peptoses are absorbed more slowly. Glucose and galactose are absorbed by active transport through the apical membranes of intestinal epitheliocytes. This process is activated by sodium transport. Glucose in the absence of sodium is transported across the membrane 100 times slower, and against a concentration gradient, glucose transport in this case ceases. Glucose accumulates in intestinal epitheleocytes and is subsequently transported across basolateral membranes into the intercellular fluid and blood along a concentration gradient. Fructose absorption is independent of sodium transport and is active. The possibility of passive fructose transport through the apical membranes of epitheliocytes is not excluded. Various factors, especially internal secretion glands, are involved in the regulation of carbohydrate absorption in the small intestine. Glucose absorption is enhanced by hormones of the adrenal, pituitary, thyroid and pancreatic glands. Increase the absorption of glucose serotonin and acetylcholine. Somewhat slows down this process histamine, and somatostatin significantly inhibits. Absorbed monosaccharides in the intestine through the portal vein system enter the liver. Here, a significant portion is retained and converted into glycogen. Part of the glucose enters the general bloodstream and spreads throughout the body and is used as a source of energy. Some of the glucose is converted into triglycerides and stored in fat depots.

Glucose absorption is enhanced by adrenal, pituitary, thyroid hormones, as well as serotonin and acetylcholine. Somatostatin and, to a lesser extent, histamine inhibit glucose absorption.

Absorption of lipid hydrolysis products. Fats, or lipids, are represented in food products in the form of triglycerides (glycerol and 3 fatty acids), phospholipids (glycerol, fatty acid, phosphoric acid and amino alcohols), glycolipids (glycerol, fatty acid and carbohydrates), cholesterol and steroids. In general, about 80-100 g of fats are needed per day, of which 30% are of vegetable origin, as they contain essential amino acids (linoleic and linolenic). Hydrolysis of fat occurs due to pancreatic and intestinal lipase, as well as phospholipase. Lipase activity is increased by colipase, a factor that binds to lipase and increases its activity. Calcium ions also increase lipase activity. The action of lipases results in the formation of a mixture of fatty acids, glycerol mono-, di- and triglycerides. Further from this mixture, and with the participation of bile acids, phospholipids and cholesterol, tiny droplets - *micelles* - are formed. Absorption of fats depends on their emulsification and hydrolysis and is most active in the 12-intestine and the proximal part of the jejunum. As a result of the action of enzymes (lipase and phospholipase), diglycerides are formed from triglycerides, followed by monoglycerides and fatty acids. Absorption of micelles is accomplished as follows:

1) their transport from the intestinal cavity to the apical membrane of intestinal epitheliocytes, carried out with the help of bile acids. In this case, bile acids remain in the intestinal cavity and are absorbed in the ileum by the mechanism of active transport;

2) their passage through the apical membrane into the enterocyte with subsequent disintegration of micelles and synthesis of human-specific triglycerides;

3) the passage of triglycerides through the endoplasmic network of epitheliocytes and the conversion of triglycerides into *chylomicrons* - tiny fat particles consisting of triglycerides, cholesterol, phospholipids and globulins, encased in a thin protein shell;

4) chylomicrons leave the epitheliocytes through the basolateral membranes, passing into the connective tissue spaces of the villi;

5) passage of chylomicron into the central lymphatic vessel of the villi, this is facilitated by the contraction of villi due to vilikinin. The main amount of fat is absorbed into the lymph and 3-4 hours after a meal, the lymphatic vessels are filled with a large amount of lymph, resembling milk and called milky juice.

Under normal conditions, a small amount of fat absorbed in the intestine, represented by triglycerides of fatty acids, whose molecules contain short hydrocarbon chains, enters the blood. Water-soluble glycerol can also be transported into the blood capillaries from epitheliocytes and intercellular space. The formation of chylomicrons in epitheliocytes is not necessary for the absorption of fats whose molecules contain short and medium hydrocarbon chains. Small amounts of chylomicrons may enter the blood vessels of villi.

The rate of lipid absorption is regulated by the nervous system: parasympathetic nerves speed it up and sympathetic nerves slow it down. In addition, hormones of the adrenal cortex, thyroid gland, pituitary gland, and the 12th intestine (secretin and cholicystokinin) stimulate lipid absorption.

Absorption of water and mineral salts. Most water is absorbed into the blood, and a small amount is absorbed into the lymph. Water absorption begins in the stomach, but most intensively in the small intestine. Absorption of water is carried out along an osmotic gradient. Most water absorption is conjugated by the transport of sodium ions, chlorine, sugars, and amino acids. Inhibition of water absorption is realized in the absence of bile, vagotomy. Of the hormones weaken water absorption gastrin, secretin, cholicystokinin. ACTH enhances absorption of water and chlorides, thyroxine enhances absorption of water, glucose and lipids.

Sodium is intensively absorbed in the small intestine and ileum. Sodium entry into the epitheliocyte is carried out passively by an electrochemical gradient. From epitheliocytes, sodium ions are actively transported through basolateral membranes into the intercellular fluid, blood, and lymph. In the small intestine, the transport of sodium ions is coupled with chloride ions. In the large intestine there is an exchange of absorbed sodium ions for potassium ion. The absorption of sodium ions is enhanced by pituitary and adrenal hormones, and inhibited by gastrin, secretin and cholicystokinin.

Absorption of potassium ions occurs mainly in the small intestine via passive transport along an electrochemical gradient.

Absorption of chlorine ions occurs in the stomach, and most actively in the ileum by the mechanism of active and passive transport.

Of the divalent cations absorbed in the intestine, calcium, magnesium, zinc, copper and iron ions are the most important.

Calcium is absorbed along the entire length of the gastrointestinal tract, but is most actively absorbed in the colon and jejunum. Magnesium, zinc and iron ions are absorbed in the same section. Absorption of copper occurs predominantly in the stomach. In the process of calcium absorption, the mechanisms of facilitated and simple diffusion are involved. It is believed that there is a calcium pump in the basal membrane of enterocytes, which ensures that calcium is pumped out of the cell into the blood against an electrochemical gradient. Calcium absorption is stimulated by bile. Absorption of magnesium, zinc and copper is by passive absorption. Iron absorption is accomplished passively and actively. When iron enters the enterocyte, it combines with apoferritin, resulting in the formation of the metalloprotein ferritin, which is the major depot of iron in the body.

Vitamin absorption. Water-soluble vitamins (C, riboflavin) are absorbed by diffusion. Vitamin B_{12} is absorbed in the ileum. Absorption of fat-soluble vitamins (A, D, E, K) is closely associated with fat absorption.

Lecture 22.

<u>Topic: Food motivation. Physiological basis of hunger and satiety.</u>

The aim is to know the physiologic mechanisms of food motivation formation.

The objectives are.

(a) Uncover theories of food motivation;

b) show the digestive center and its structure;

c) to consider food motivation from the perspective of functional systems of the organism

Content:

Hunger is a subjective expression of the body's nutritional needs. Subjective manifestation of hunger are: nausea, feelings of "sucking under the spoon" (burning, pressure and pain in the epigastric region - hunger pains), headache, dizziness, feeling of general weakness. The objective external manifestation of hunger is a behavioral reaction aimed at eliminating hunger - searching for and eating food (*food motivation*) with overcoming all sorts of, even significant obstacles. Emotional feeling of hunger in the form of subjective manifestations is connected with the activity of limbic structures and the cortex of the large hemispheres. When feeling hunger, there is an increase in the motor activity of the stomach and the 12-pronged intestine, opening of the pyloric sphincter, which is a manifestation of the periodic activity of the digestive tract (increased activity during 30 min every 90 min). The physiological significance of "hunger" periodic activity consists in maintaining homeostasis of the organism by means of transition from exogenous to endogenous type of nutrition. The state of hunger is also characterized by a certain decrease in the intensity of metabolic processes in tissues and a decrease in the concentration of a number of nutrients in the blood due to which the "hungry" blood is formed, as well as periodic emptying of nutrient depots (mainly carbohydrates and fats) from the liver, muscle tissue and fatty fiber.

Close to the concept of hunger is the concept of *appetite*. Appetite (from Latin - appetito aspiration, desire) is an emotional feeling associated with the desire to eat. Appetite is based on the formation of needs and motivations, so appetite is formed on the basis of excitations of neurons of the cortex of the large hemispheres and the limbic system. Appetite, in contrast to hunger, is the desire to eat certain food depending on the initial need, national and individual habits (hunger - the desire to eat any food). It has now been established that in the mucosa of the 12th *perestine is* formed a hormone of peptide nature - *arenterin,* which reduces appetite.

Appetite disorder. *Anorexia* is a sharp decrease in appetite up to absence of appetite. It is associated with pathology of the hunger center and, probably, with disruption of the neurons of the cerebral cortex and limbic system. *Bulemia* (from Greek - bull hunger) - a sharp increase in appetite. It is also associated with a violation of the structures of the food center. *Perversion of appetite* - there is a need to take with food inedible substances (ash, earth, coal, kerosene, paper, etc.). In some cases - it is the result of a lack of certain substances in the body, in other cases - a manifestation of mental disorder (eating feces - coprophagia). At the heart of perverted appetite are disorders of the neurons of the food center.

Subjective and objective manifestations of hunger and appetite are caused by excitation of neurons in various parts of the CNS: in the cerebral cortex, in the limbic system, reticular formation and hypothalamus. Together these neurons constitute the *food center*. The leading section (peutzmecker), from which the activation of the entire food center spreads, are the *lateral nuclei of the hypothalamus*. Irritation of these nuclei leads to increased food intake, and their destruction leads to food refusal. These hypothalamic nuclei are called the *hunger center*. When the *ventro-medial nuclei of the* hypothalamus are irritated, food refusal (aphagia) occurs, and when they are destroyed, increased food intake (bulimia, hyperphagia) occurs. These hypothalamic nuclei are called the *satiety center*. Satiety occurs before the absorption of products of hydrolysis of nutrients. In this regard, there are two types of satiety: primary, or sensory, and secondary, or metabolic (nutritive).

Sensory satiation occurs as a result of afferent flow of impulses coming from various receptors of the mouth, stomach, excited by the ingested food. The conditioned reflex process is also of great importance to the processes of sensory satiation. Previous experience with a particular type of food allows a person to evaluate its caloric and plastic effects. Secondary satiation occurs much later, when the products of hydrolysis begin to enter the blood. This is approximately 1.5 to 2 hours from the time of ingestion. Currently, there are several theories that explain the occurrence of hunger and food motivation with subsequent satiation.

The glucostatic theory, according to which the sensation of hunger is associated with a decrease in blood glucose. Apparently, there are glucoreceptors in the hypothalamus that perceive changes in blood glucose. This is confirmed experimentally: during intravenous injection of glucose, the electrical activity of neurons of the lateral nucleus (hunger center) decreases and the activity of ventromedial nuclei (satiety center) increases.

The aminoacidostatic theory, according to which the excitation of the hunger center is accomplished by a decrease in amino acids in the blood.

Lipostatic theory, according to which the stimulus of the hunger center is the lack of metabolites formed when fat is mobilized from its depots. It is believed that the excitation of the hunger center is carried out by signals from fat depots when fat is released from them.

The thermostatic theory, suggests the suppression of the hunger center as a result of the increase in the temperature of the blood that bathes it, which occurs during the ingestion of food.

The hydrostatic theory connects the emergence of hunger with the body's water resources - a decrease in water supply (about 8 liters of water is released into the digestive cavity when eating) causes inhibition of the hunger center.

Metabolic theory - this theory was proposed by academician A.M. Ugolev. According to this theory, the main reason for the excitation of the hunger center is the lack of intermediate products of the Krebs cycle, which are common in the oxidation of nutrients (proteins, fats and carbohydrates).

It has now been established that in natural conditions the state of the food center is determined both by the composition of the chemical composition of the blood and by nerve impulses from digestive organs, nutrient depots, numerous intero- and extero-receptors, as well as from the centers of many reflexes. Thus, excitation of the hunger center occurs primarily due to the body's internal need for food intake due to a lack of Krebs cycle intermediates (metabolic theory). Humoral excitation of the hunger center causes a special activity of the digestive tract ("hunger" periodic activity), resulting in an increased flow of afferent impulses to the hunger center, which leads to mobilization of the fat depot (the transition from exogenous to endogenous type of nutrition), which increases the flow of afferent impulses to the hunger center. As a result, there are a number of unpleasant sensations in the form of burning, pressure and pain in the epigastric region, nausea, slight dizziness - this is a subjective expression of the objective food requirement of the organism.

The process of excitation involves the limbic system and the cortex of the large hemispheres - there is *food motivation* - purposeful behavior associated with the search and ingestion of food. Food intake is accompanied by a flow of afferent impulses from mechano-, thermo- and chemoreceptors of the oral cavity and stomach to the satiety center. On the other hand, the amount of intermediate products of the Krebs cycle increases in the blood, which causes humoral excitation of the satiety center and inhibition of the hunger center - there is a refusal to eat.

Lecture 23.

<u>Topic: Metabolism of substances and energy. Accounting of energy consumption and energy input. Direct and indirect calorimetry. Classification of people according to their energy expenditure (WHO).</u>

Objective - to know the metabolism between the organism and the external environment as the basic condition of life and preservation of homeostasis, the plastic and energetic role of nutrients, the balance of their input and expenditure.

The objectives are.

a) reveal the transformation of energy in an organism (free and bound energy, entropy);

b) show the role of the basic exchange (actual and proper) and the working allowance;

c) Discover Hess's law and its significance in determining the caloric value of nutrients;

d) show the methods of accounting for energy inputs and outputs;

e) give a classification of people according to their energy expenditure.

Content:

Metabolism is a set of processes consisting of:

1) nutrient intake into the body;

2) anabolism (assimilation) - biosynthesis of organic substances, components of cells and tissues;

3) catabolism (dissimilation) - cleavage of complex molecules of cell components;

4) release of energy and end products of decomposition. The predominance of anabolic processes provides growth, accumulation of

body weight, while the predominance of catabolic processes leads to partial destruction of tissue structures, reduction of body weight. Metabolism is accompanied by energy conversion, the transition of potential chemical energy into kinetic energy (mainly mechanical and partly electrical). To compensate for the energy expenditure of the body, to maintain body weight and meet the needs of growth, it is necessary to receive nutrients with energy potential (proteins, fats and carbohydrates), vitamins, mineral salts and water from the external environment. This is achieved through nutrition. On the other hand, it is necessary that the body is cleansed from the end products of decay, which are formed during the breakdown of various substances. This is accomplished by the work of the excretory organs. Thus in the process of metabolism, complex organic substances with a high energy content are transformed into less complex substances, and energy is released, which is transferred from one type to another. The energy released in the organism can be determined and expressed in units of heat - calories. The method of determining the amount of energy formed in the body is called *calorimetry*.

The kilojoule (kJ) is taken as the unit of energy: 1 kcal equals 4.19 kJ. In addition, such units as kcal/min, kcal/hour, kcal/day are used. The unit kcal/day is usually used to estimate the value of basic metabolism, and kcal/min or kcal/hour is used to estimate energy expenditure in production activities, sports, and everyday life. To compare energy expenditure in different individuals, the normalized units of kcal/kg body weight per unit time or $kcal/m^2$ body surface area per unit time are used. The Committee of Experts on Physical Activity of Exchange (FAO) and WHO recommends the use of units that are multiples of the basic exchange rate (BER). For example, under conditions of physiologic rest, a subject's energy expenditure is 1700 kcal/day and under conditions of physical activity 3400 kcal/day, i.e., 2BOO.

Energy conversion in the body occurs as follows:

1) during oxidation of proteins, fats and carbohydrates, a part of energy is converted into chemical energy and is accumulated in the body in the form of ATP, another part of energy is converted into heat - *primary heat.* Further, when ATP is broken down, the energy is used for *basic metabolism (WM), work gain (WG), the* rest is often converted into heat - *secondary heat.* Consequently, the amount of heat generated in the organism becomes a measure of the total energy of chemical bonds subjected to biological oxidation and can be expressed in units of heat - calories or joules. From the point of view of thermodynamics, there is free energy (it can be used for work) and bound, or depreciated energy, which cannot be used to do useful work because it is degraded. In closed systems, all free energy spontaneously changes to bound energy and so these systems become inoperable. The human body is an open thermodynamic system. It constantly receives a flow of free energy. At the same time it gives bound energy to the environment. Due to these two flows, the entropy of a living organism (the degree of disorder, chaos, degradation) remains at a constant (minimum) level. If the flow of free energy (not entropy) decreases or the flow of bound energy (entropy) increases, the total entropy of the organism increases, which can lead to its thermodynamic death. Thus, according to the thermodynamics of living systems, life is a struggle with entropy. Free energy for the organism can come with nutrients that have energy potential (proteins, fats and carbohydrates). It should be noted that during the hydrolysis of nutrients in the gastrointestinal tract, a small portion of free energy (less than 0.5%) is released. This energy cannot be used for useful work, as it is not accumulated by macroergamy such as ATP. It is converted into heat energy, which is used to maintain temperature homeostasis. The main stage of energy release in the body (94.5%) is carried out in the Krebs

cycle. The major part of this free energy (52-55%) manages to accumulate into macroergic energy (ATP). The remaining part is lost as primary heat as a result of the "imperfection" of biological oxidation.

The energy value of nutrients can be determined by burning them in a special vessel (Bertloh calorimetric bomb). This produces carbon dioxide and water with the release of heat, which is accounted for by the degree of heating of the water. It is established that burning 1 g of nutrients in a calorimetric bomb generates energy: burning 1 g of protein - 5.4 kcal; burning 1 g of fat - 9.3 kcal; burning 1 g of carbohydrates - 4.1 kcal. These values are called the *caloric value of nutrients* (energy that is released when burning 1 g of nutrients). In the conditions of the body (biological oxidation occurs), the caloric value of carbohydrates and fats is the same as in a calorimetric bomb, since the oxidation of these substances in the body is carried out to carbon dioxide and water. According to Hess's law, the amount of heat released by nutrients does not depend on the intermediate reactions, but on the initial and final products. For protein in the conditions of the body, the caloric value is lower than in the bomb and is 4.1 kcal, since protein in the body is not completely oxidized and part of it leaves the body in the form of urea, ammonia, ammonium. The values of the energy value of nutrients are used to determine the energy intake. For this purpose, it is also necessary to know the amount of nutrients used in grams, which is determined by special tables.

Basic metabolic energy (BME) is the energy that the body expends under three standard conditions: 1) muscular rest (a person is lying down for 20-30 min); 2) in conditions of comfort temperature at $+20+22^0$ C (in this case the body does not expend energy to maintain temperature homeostasis); 3) on an empty stomach (12-14 hours after the last meal), in order not to take into account energy expenditure associated with the digestion of nutrients. In women, due to the absence of high levels of androgens, GS is 10 - 15% less than in men. GS is consumed for ventricular systole, the act of breathing, processes occurring in the nephron and assimilation processes in all cells. According to data provided by WHO (1987) the energy of the GS is expended on: liver - 27%, brain - 19%, heart - 7%, kidneys - 10%, muscles - 18%, other organs - 19%. "Other" includes energy expenditure for thermoregulation. AO depends on sex, age, and body size. The value of GS per unit of body weight is maximum in newborns and infants, and later on GS gradually decreases, especially after 20-25 years of age.

Working gain is the energy that is expended for: 1) assimilation of nutrients - specific dynamic action of food (SDDP); 2) for all kinds of activities - performing muscular and mental work, carrying out respiration, digestion, blood circulation, maintaining body temperature, overcoming osmotic forces during secretory and excretory processes, etc.

Direct calorimetry. Direct calorimetry is based on the direct accounting in biocalorimeters of the amount of heat released by the organism. A biocalorimeter is a sealed and well-insulated chamber. Water circulates in the chamber through tubes. The heat generated by a human or animal in the chamber heats the circulating water. From the amount of water flowing and the change in its temperature, the amount of heat released by the organism is calculated. The method of direct calorimetry is very complex. Taking into account that the basis of heat formation in the body are oxidative processes that consume oxygen and form CO_2 it is possible to use indirect, indirect determination of heat formation in the body by its gas exchange.

Indirect calorimetry. This method takes into account the amount of oxygen consumed and carbon dioxide released and then calculates the energy expenditure of the body. Thus, to determine the energy expenditure of the organism by indirect calorimetry it is necessary to know the following:

1) the amount of oxygen consumed by the body;

2) caloric equivalent of oxygen - the amount of heat released after the body consumes 1 liter of oxygen. Oxygen absorbed by the body is used to oxidize proteins, fats and carbohydrates. The oxidation of 1 g of each of these substances requires different amounts of oxygen. It has been found that when 1 liter of oxygen is absorbed, different amounts of energy are released depending on which substances are used for oxidation: proteins - 19.26 kJ (4.6 kcal), fats - 19.64 kJ (4.69 kcal), carbohydrates - 21.14 kJ (5.05 kcal); 3) released carbon dioxide;

3) respiratory quotient (RQ) - the ratio of released carbon dioxide to absorbed oxygen. According to this indicator it is possible to determine at oxidation of which substances energy expenditures of the organism took place. DK is different for oxidation of proteins, fats and carbohydrates: for carbohydrates - 1; for proteins - 0.8; for fats - 0.7. In a mixed diet in humans, DK is 0.85 - 0.89.

Basic metabolism. The value of basal metabolism depends on body weight and body surface area. On average, in men, GS is 4.19 kJ (1kcal) per 1 kg of body weight per hour, or 7117 kJ (1700 kcal) per day. In women of the same mass (70 kg) and height (165 cm), it is 10 to 15% lower. The AO intensity per 1 kg of body weight in children is much higher than in adults. If we recalculate the AO intensity per 1 kg of body weight, it turns out that it is different in warm-blooded animals of different species and in people with different body weight and height. If we recalculate the AO intensity per 1 m^2 of body surface, the AO values obtained in different animals and humans do not differ so sharply.

A distinction is made between the proper value of the basic metabolism (BEP) and the actual value (BEP). The BEM is determined by special tables of Harris-Benedict, for which it is necessary to know gender, weight, height and age. There are two versions of these tables, one for men and one for women. The FAO/WHO expert report provides formulas for calculating BAF, which have been obtained in recent years from a study of a large population of people depending on age in kcal/day: 0-3 years 60.9MT-54 (men) and 61MT-51 (women); 3-10 years 22.7MT+495 and 22.5MT+499; 10-18 years 17.5MT+651 and 12.2MT+746; 18-30 years 15.3MT+679 and 14.7MT+496; 30-60 years 11.6MT+879 and 8.7MT+829; over 60 years 13.5MT+487 and 10.5MT+596, where MT is body mass in kg. OLF is determined by direct or indirect calorimetry under three standard conditions. The ratio of OLF to DOO, expressed as a percentage, is then determined. In the norm, this value corresponds to $100 \pm 10\%$. This ratio of more than 110% indicates thyroid hyperfunction, and less than 90% indicates hypofunction.

Physical activity significantly increases energy expenditure, so the daily energy expenditure of a healthy person who spends part of the day in movement and physical work significantly exceeds the GS value. This increase in energy expenditure constitutes the working gain: it is the greater the more intensive the muscle work. The degree of energy expenditure at different physical activity is determined by the *physical activity factor (PAF)*, which is the ratio of total energy expenditure per day to the value of the GS. This index varies with different activities (based on kcal/min): walking, washing, dressing, short-term standing posture - 1.4; singing and dancing - 3.2; washing clothes - 2.2; walking around the house - 2.5; slow walks in the street - 2.8; playing cards - 1.4; cooking - 1.8; daily cleaning - 2.7; office work - 1.3; bricklaying - 3.3; carpentry - 2.8; working with pitchforks - 6.8; hunting and fishing - 3.4; hand milking cows - 2.9; loading sacks on a wheelbarrow - 7.4. According to this principle, the male population is divided into five groups: 1) workers engaged in predominantly mental labor (9799 - 10265 kJ, or 2100 - 2450 kcal; CFA - 1.4); 2) workers engaged in light physical labor (10475 - 11732 kJ, or 2500 - 2800 kcal; CFA - 1.6); 3) workers engaged in moderate labor (12360 - 13827 kJ, or 2950 - 3300 kcal; CFA - 1.9); 4) workers engaged in heavy physical labor (14246 - 16131 kJ, or 3400 - 3850 kcal; CFA - 2.2); 5) workers engaged in especially heavy physical labor (16131 - 17598 kJ, or 3850 - 4200 kcal; CFA - 2.5). The fifth group is noted only in men. Differences in body energy expenditures in the groups depend on sex (more in men), age (decreasing after 40 years), degree of recreation activity and level of public services. The female population is divided into four groups by energy expenditures.

According to FAO/WHO experts, there are only three categories of labor severity: light, medium and heavy. At the same time, energy expenditures expressed in multiples of GS are equal: light labor - 1.7OO for men and women; medium labor - 2.7OO for men and 2.2OO for women; heavy labor - 3.8OO for men and 2.8OO for women.

Daily energy consumption of children and adolescents depends on age: 6 months - 1 year - 3349 kJ, or 800 kcal; 1 - 1.5 years - 5443 (1300); 1.5 - 2 years - 6280 (1500); 3 - 4 years - 7536 (1800); 5 - 6 years - 8374 (2000); 7 - 10 years - 10048 (2400); 11 - 14 years - 11932 (2850); 14 - 17 years (boys) - 13188 (3150), (girls) - 11514 (2750). In old age, energy expenditure decreases and by the age of 80 years is 8373 - 9211 kJ (2000 - 2200 kcal).

The value of total metabolism reflects the degree of physical activity of a person. If it is low - 2400 - 3500 kcal / day, it indicates hypodynamia. This condition is dangerous for health: against this background, the risk of early onset of atherosclerosis, coronary heart disease, peptic ulcer disease of the stomach and 12-pearl intestine, etc. increases. Long-term observations of the American doctor Cooper showed that the frequency of diseases and mortality from them depends on the level of physical activity: 1) mortality from all causes at low mobility is 64 per 10000 population in men, 140 in women, at moderate mobility 26/16, maximum mobility 20/7; 2) mortality from cardiovascular diseases at low mobility 25/7, at moderate mobility - 8/3 and at maximum mobility 7/10; 3) mortality from cancer - at low mobility - 20/16, at moderate mobility - 3/1, at maximum mobility - 5/1. Japanese researchers say that a person should walk about 10 kilometers per day on foot or about 5-7 kilometers in the form of light jogging. Russian physiologists believe that the norm is 3.33 kcal/min, or 4,795 kcal/day. According to FAO/WHO (1987) for maintenance of high working capacity each person needs daily 20 minutes of physical activity with intensity of 4-5 kcal/min, or 5OO. Thus, physical activity of modern man is one of the important problems of longevity and low morbidity.

Specific dynamic effect of food - after a meal, the intensity of metabolism and energy expenditure of the organism increases compared to the level in the conditions of OO. The increase in energy expenditure begins one hour after a meal and reaches its maximum in 3 hours and remains at this level for several hours. SDDP is highest with protein food (30% of the GS), lowest with carbohydrate food (5%), and 12-14% with fat intake.

Regulation of energy metabolism. The level of energy metabolism is closely dependent on physical activity, emotional stress, the nature of nutrition, the degree of tension of thermoregulation and other factors. Numerous data testify to the participation of the cortex of the large hemispheres in the regulation of energy metabolism: 1) conditionally reflex change in oxygen consumption and energy exchange (any previously indifferent stimulus, associated in time with muscle activity, can serve as a signal to increase metabolism; increase in energy exchange in an athlete before the start); 2) a subject under hypnosis can increase or decrease energy exchange. The hypothalamus plays a special role in the regulation of energy exchange. Here regulatory influences are formed, which are realized by autonomic nerves or humoral link due to changes in secretion of a number of endocrine glands: thyroid hormones (thyroxine and triiodothyronine) and hormones of the brain layer of adrenal glands (adrenaline, noradrenaline) significantly increase energy expenditure of the organism.

PHYSIOLOGICAL BASIS OF NUTRITION

Nutrition - the process of intake, digestion, absorption and assimilation in the body of food substances (nutrients) necessary to cover the plastic and energy needs of the body, the formation of physiologically active substances. There is a distinction between *natural and artificial* nutrition (clinical parenteral and probe enteral). Also distinguished therapeutic and therapeutic and preventive. Food substances include, first of all, proteins, fats and carbohydrates, the oxidation of which releases a certain amount of heat in the body (for fat - 9.3 kcal/g, or 37 kJ/g, for proteins and carbohydrates - 4.1 kcal/g, or 17 kJ/g). According to the *rule of isodynamics*, they can be mutually substituted in meeting the energy needs of the body. However, each of food substances and their fragments has specific plastic properties and properties of biologically active substances. Substitution of some substances in the diet by others leads to disruption of body functions.

The biological value of nutrients is determined by the presence of essential components in them. The *biological value of* animal proteins is higher than that of vegetable proteins. The digestibility of proteins of animal origin is on average 97%, and vegetable proteins - 83-85%. For reliable stability of nitrogen balance it is recommended to take 85-90 g of proteins with food (at least 1 g of protein per 1 kg of body weight). The biological value of dietary lipids is determined by the presence of essential fatty acids, the ability to digest and absorption in the digestive tract (assimilation). Butter and pork fat are digested by 93-98%, beef fat by 80-94%, sunflower oil by 86-90%, margarine by 94-98%. The main amount of carbohydrates enters the body in the form of polysaccharides of plant foods. After hydrolysis and absorption, carbohydrates are used to meet energy needs. On average, a person consumes 400 - 500 g of carbohydrates per day, of which 350-400 g is starch, 50 - 100 g mono- and disaccharides. Excess carbohydrates are stored as fat.

The daily water requirement in an adult is 21-43 ml/kg. Insufficient water intake causes dehydration of the body, which has a different degree of severity depending on the level of dehydration. Death occurs when 1/3 - 1/4 of the total amount of water in the body is lost, which accounts for 60% of body weight.

The starting material for the renewal and creation of living tissue and the source of energy is food. Human nutrition should be *rational*. It should meet the needs of the body in plastic substances and energy (this is achieved by the consumption of nutrients - proteins, fats and carbohydrates), mineral salts, vitamins and water, to ensure normal vital activity of the body, good health, high efficiency and resistance to infection, proper growth and development of children's bodies.

The following principles should be followed to follow a sound diet:

1) the caloric content of the food ration should cover the energy expenditure of the organism, which is determined by the type of labor activity;

2) the possibility of using the law of *isodynamics, i.e. the* interchangeability of proteins, fats and carbohydrates to cover the energy expenditures of the organism. For example, 1 g of fat, in terms of its

caloric value, can be replaced by 2.3 g of protein or carbohydrates. However, it should be noted that nutrients, in addition to their energy function, have a plastic function (used to build new cells);

3) the diet should contain the optimal amount of proteins, fats and carbohydrates for a given group of workers. Protein content in the daily ration has a special place. On the sufficiency or insufficiency of protein ration can judge the *nitrogen balance*: the correspondence of the amount of nitrogen introduced with food, the amount of nitrogen excreted from the body. In the norm there should be a *nitrogen balance* - a state in which the amount of nitrogen introduced into the body is equal to the amount of nitrogen excreted from the body. If the protein diet is insufficient, there is a state of *negative nitrogen balance* - less nitrogen is introduced into the body than is excreted with breakdown products. This condition occurs during starvation, severe infectious diseases, in old age, during tumor decay, etc.

Positive nitrogen balance is a condition when more nitrogen is supplied to the body than is excreted, i.e. nitrogen retention in the body. This condition is observed during the growth of the organism, during pregnancy, after prolonged fasting, after severe infectious diseases, during tumor growth;

4) the optimal ratio of proteins, fats and carbohydrates - b : w : y = 1 : 1,2 : 3,6 should be observed in the food ration;

5) the food ration should fully satisfy the body's need for vitamins, mineral salts and water;

6) it is recommended to include in the food ration one third of the daily norm of proteins and fats of animal origin;

7) when observing the energy balance of the body, it is necessary to take into account the degree of assimilation of various nutrients;

8) foods rich in protein (meat, fish, legumes) are recommended to be consumed during the daytime hours, in the evening - dairy and vegetable dishes;

9) adherence to a proper diet, which includes: a) regularity of eating at the same time - this contributes to the conditionally-reflexive release of gastric juice, which I.P. Pavlov called "priming". The function of this juice is to prepare the digestive organs for the reception of food; b) fractional feeding - food should enter the gastrointestinal tract in small portions. The most optimal is considered four meals at the same time the most rational is the following distribution of food: breakfast - 20-25%, second breakfast - 10-15%, lunch - 40-45%, dinner - 20-25%. With three meals a day: breakfast 25-30%, lunch - 45-50%, dinner - 20-25%. With a tendency to obesity is recommended more frequent meals (while the caloric content should not exceed the norm) - 5-6 times. With frequent meals, the excitability of the center of hunger decreases, and the excitability of the center of satiety increases, which reduces appetite; c) the time between breakfast and lunch, as well as between lunch and dinner at three meals a day should be 5-6 hours; d) the use of dinner should be no later than 2-3 hours before bedtime;

10) the diet should include 10-15% of ballast substances (dietary fiber): polysaccharides such as cellulose, hemicellulose, pectin, lignin. In large quantities, ballast substances are found in vegetables, fruits and cereals. They enhance intestinal motor function, serve as food for microorganisms of the large intestine. Ballast substances increase glucose tolerance, modify glucose absorption, reduce blood cholesterol levels and have antitoxic properties;

11) a certain amount of vitamins and mineral salts should be included in the diet.

Theories of nutrition. Each organism combines biochemical traits unique to it and traits common to that biological group. This means that there is no ideal diet (diet and nutritional regimen). Each person needs an individual set of components of the diet that meets the individual characteristics of his metabolism. However, at the present stage of development of science and practice, an individualized diet cannot be implemented. At present, two main theories are guided in the compilation of food ration.

Balanced nutrition. Balanced nutrition is characterized by the optimal correspondence of the amount and ratios of all components of food to the physiological needs of the body. This theory assumes compliance with a number of principles in the preparation of the food ration: 1) the food taken, taking into account its digestibility, should replenish the energy expenditure of the body, which is defined as the sum of the basic metabolism, the specific dynamic action of food and energy expenditure for the work performed. It should be noted that if the daily requirement is regularly exceeded, 100 g of muffin bun leads to the accumulation of 15-30 g of fat in the human body, which during the year can lead to the deposition of 5.4-10.8 kg of fat in the depot; 2) the food ration should be balanced proteins, fats and carbohydrates. The average ratio of their mass is 1:1,2:3,6 (1:1,2:4), energy value - 15:30:55%. This ratio satisfies the energy and plastic needs of the body; 2) should be optimized proteins with essential and substitutable amino acids, fats with different saturation of fatty acids, as well as the optimal ratio of products of animal and vegetable origin; 3) the presence of vitamins and minerals in the diet; 4) regularity of meals at the same time of day. With three meals a day it is advisable to distribute the daily ration by energy value as follows: breakfast - 25-30%, lunch - 45-50%, dinner - 20-25%. The time between breakfast and lunch, lunch and dinner is 5-6 hours, between dinner and sleep 3-4 hours.

According to academician A.M. Ugolev, there were several serious errors in the theory of balanced nutrition:

1) improved food was created - when food products were enriched with substances directly involved in metabolism, ballast and harmful substances were removed from the products at the same time. That is why modern bread, cereals, oil, sugar, salt, rice are refined. The use of refined products has led to the development of diseases of civilization (myocardial infarction, hypertension, atherosclerosis, varicose veins, thrombosis, chronic bronchitis, pulmonary emphysema, gastrointestinal diseases, multiple sclerosis, diabetes);

2) direct nutrition (parenteral), the idea of which was formulated by the French chemist P. Bertlo in 1908, proved to be suitable only in exceptional cases (in appropriate diseases), and in real everyday life its use is dangerous, because such nutrition is observed dysbacteriosis - the development of pathogenic flora of microorganisms in the intestine. On the basis of the above, Ugolev A.M. proposed the theory of adequate nutrition.

Adequate nutrition. According to this theory, as well as the theory of balanced nutrition, it should fully replenish the energy and plastic needs of the body. According to the theory of adequate nutrition, the necessary components of food are not only nutrients, but also ballast substances. Normal nutrition is conditioned not by a single flow of nutrients from the gastrointestinal tract, but by several flows of nutritive and regulatory substances of vital importance. According to this theory, there is an endecology of the host organism, which is formed by the microflora of its intestine. The balance of nutrients is achieved as a result of the release of nutrients from food structures during enzymatic breakdown of its molecules due to cavity and membrane digestion, as well as due to the synthesis of new substances, including essential ones.

Flows of substances. According to M.A. Ugolev, the following flows are distinguished:

1) nutrients from food;

2) ballast;

3) hormones and other physiologically active substances. For example, it has been found that the breakdown of milk and wheat proteins produces morphine-like substances - exorphins, which act similarly to endorphins;

4) three streams of bacterial metabolites: a) a stream of nutrients modified by microorganisms (e.g., amine stream), b) a stream of secondary nutrients - useful substances that are released from nutrients with the participation of microorganisms (e.g., amino acids, carbohydrates, fats), c) a stream of products of microbial activity;

5) The flow of substances coming in with contaminated food.

Endoecology. According to the theory of balanced nutrition, repopulating the gastrointestinal tract with microorganisms is undesirable and harmful. It turns out that microorganisms are necessary and beneficial. Suppression of microorganisms (when prescribing antibiotics) often leads to a shift in the metabolic balance of the body. According to A.M. Ugolev, in conditions of starvation it is necessary to use grass, just to support the vitality of microorganisms, because in conditions of starvation their existence is no less important than the supply of food from outside. When the microflora is disturbed (by illness, use of antibiotic therapy, stress, parenteral nutrition), dysbacteriosis occurs, which causes secondary disease.

The theory of adequate nutrition attaches great importance to the body's defense systems against the penetration of various harmful substances. From this point of view, the entry of food into the gastrointestinal tract is considered not only as a way to replenish energy and plastic materials, but also as an allergic and toxic aggression. Due to effective defense this aggression is neutralized. The following defense mechanisms are distinguished: 1) mechanical filter for large molecules-antigens - carried out due to the glycocalyx of enterocytes; 2) hydrolysis of antigens by enzymes of the gastrointestinal tract; 3) immune system of the gastrointestinal tract, which is represented by peyer's plaques of the small intestine and lymphoid tissue of the appendix. There are B- and T-lymphocytes in the gastrointestinal tract. On average, there are 6-40 lymphocytes in 100 intestinal epithelial cells.

Thus, according to the adequate theory of nutrition, the ideal food is that food which is useful to a given person under given conditions, adequate to the human condition. To determine its composition is a difficult task, but real.

Rational nutrition. Rational nutrition refers to a compromise between efficient nutrition and reality. The trade-off is generated by the scarcity of nutritious foods or their high cost.

Some ideas about other types of rational nutrition: 1) *Vegetarianism* involves eating only plant foods. The idea originated in antiquity, but was particularly developed at the end of the 1st century. A distinction is made between old-vegetarianism (using only plant foods) and young-vegetarianism (allowing the use of animal products such as milk, eggs, butter). Vegetarians believe that products of animal origin (especially meat) when hydrolyzed in the GI tract form an increased amount of putrefactive and toxic products that poison the body. On the other hand, plant products are rich in biologically active substances, vitamins, mineral salts, phytoncides, enzymes, dietary fiber, contribute to the prevention of atherosclerosis. At present it is considered that young vegetarianism in adulthood is not harmful; 2) *Cheese-eating* rejects any culinary processing of food, as thermal processing destroys valuable biologically active substances. We can agree with this principle, but it is inappropriate to extend it to all products. For example, when consuming meat, fish, poultry, which has not been cooked, it is possible infection with microorganisms and parasites; 3) active use of germinated wheat grains. They contain *auxin,* a plant growth hormone. It is believed that in all age groups it is useful to eat porridge from germinated wheat for breakfast. Wheat grains at the rate of 50-100g per serving, washed thoroughly with cold water, then put in a warm place for 24 hours, pouring water over them beforehand; they give small sprouts (1mm). These grains are ground on a meat grinder and thrown into boiling water or milk. Cook porridge or kisel. If you regularly eat porridge or kisel of germinated wheat for breakfast, you can achieve restoration of coordination of movement, increased visual acuity, improving the condition of the scalp, strengthening teeth, the appearance of almost complete immunity to colds. All these factors come after 1-2 weeks from the beginning of regular intake of germinated wheat.

Classification of food. According to the classification of one of the leading nutritional physiologists A.A. Pokrovsky, food substances are divided into *nutrients* and *non-food* substances.

Nutrients - *proteins* (peptides, essential and substituted amino acids), *carbohydrates* (polysaccharides, digestible carbohydrates), *lipids* (fats, fatty acids and substituted fatty acids - cholesterol, phospholipids); *vitamins* - water-soluble, including thiamine (B_1), riboflavin (B_2), niacin (nicotinic acid, or vitamin PP), pyridoxine (B_6), cyancobalamin (B_{12}), folacin (folic acid, or vitamin B_c), pantothenic acid (B_3), biotin (H), ascorbic acid (C); fat-soluble vitamins, including retinol (A) calciferols (D), tocopherols (E), phylloquinones (K), and vitamin-like substances, including bioflavonoids (P), pangamic acid (B_{15}), para-aminobenzoic acid (H_1), orotic acid, choline (B_4), inositol (B_8), methylmethionine-sulfonium (U), lipolic acid, carnitine (B)._T

Non-food substances: *ballast compounds* (cellulose, hemicellulose, pectin); *protective components of foodstuffs* (substances involved in the function of barrier tissues; substances that improve the neutralizing function of the liver; protective factors against microorganisms and viruses; factors that exhibit anticarcinogenic effect); *flavoring and aromatic substances, anti-food components*; *carcinogenic and toxic substances.*

Protective components of foodstuffs: 1) substances involved in ensuring the function of barrier tissues. These include vitamins A, C, P, B, E. For example, retinol and many B vitamins are necessary for the formation of structural components of mucous membranes of respiratory, urogenital tract, digestive tract, skin. In maintaining the integrity of cell membranes, ensuring the normal density of the wall of blood vessels are involved tocopherols, ascorbic acid. These vitamins, as well as lecithin, kephalin, sulfur-containing amino acids, citric acid, etc. exhibit the properties of antioxidants - extinguish lipid peroxidation, protecting tissues from the appearance of free radicals, which is important in stress, ionizing radiation, the presence of industrial hazards; 2) compounds that improve the neutralizing function of the liver. These compounds provide the processes of hydroxylation, methylation of toxic substances in the liver. The source of mobile methyl groups are methionine, vitamins U, B_{15}, B_{12}, choline, lecithin. For normal liver function it is necessary to receive lipotropic substances with food (substances involved in the oxidation of lipids to end products - vitamin PP, B_2, C, P, lipoic acid, lecithin, choline, potassium ions, extreme unsaturated fatty acids), preventing the accumulation of lipids in the liver; 3) substances involved in the protection of the body from microorganisms and viruses - phytoncides. For example, the juice of Antonov apples is bactericidal against dysentery bacillus. Phytoncides are not digested by the body, but pass through the entire GI tract, neutralizing microorganisms. Phytoncides are found in mustard, horseradish, garlic, onions, parsley, cabbage, beets, carrots, citrus fruits, sea buckthorn, red and black currants, strawberries, cranberries, cranberries, cranberries; 4) substances that exhibit anticarcinogenic effects - retinol, protecting the oral cavity, GI tract, bladder; a complex of ascorbic acid, tocopherol, retinol and cysteine, which inhibits the formation in the body of nitrosamines formed from precursors contained in sausage. Nitrosamines are powerful carcinogens; vitamin K and sources containing it (carrots, cabbage); ballast substances that prevent the development of colon cancer. Sources of protective substances are: milk, cottage cheese, lactic acid products, lean varieties of meat and fish in boiled form, egg white, vegetable oils, bread made of coarse flour, bran, oatmeal and buckwheat cereals, beets, carrots, pumpkin, cabbage, black currants, gooseberries, sea buckthorn, rose hips, citrus fruits. It should be noted that food products may contain substances that counteract the manifestation of the positive effects of protective substances: products rich in cholesterol - fats in large quantities, coffee and tea (caffeine causes mobilization of fat from fat depots, so the next portion of fat is again synthesized from carbohydrates in the depot); substances containing high concentrations of biogenic amines (tyramine, norepinephrine, dopamine, serotonin) - these are many types of cheese (cheddar, Roquefort, Stilton), chocolate, pineapples, tomatoes, red wines.

Anti-nutritional substances that have no toxicity, but block or inhibit the absorption of nutrients. They include: *anti-enzymes* -

substances that block pepsin, trypsin, alpha-amylase. They are found in cheese, legumes, egg white, wheat, barley. They are destroyed by heat treatment; *reducing carbohydrates* - compounds that block the digestion or metabolism of some. During heat treatment, these substances combine with amino acids (mainly leucine) and bind them, preventing their absorption (Maillard reaction); *antivitamins* substances that destroy vitamins or prevent their absorption. For vitamin B_1 antivitamin is the enzyme thiaminase, contained in raw fish, for biotin - protein avidin, contained in raw eggs; *demineralizing* substances - oxalic acid, phytin, tannins. They bind certain divalent and trivalent compounds and render them indigestible. For example, in sorrel, rhubarb the amount of oxalic acid is so high that it counteracts the absorption of calcium.

Components of food that adversely affect the body. Foods and beverages may contain: *natural toxic compounds - lectins, non-protein amino acids, glycosides* etc. *Lectins* are glycoproteins that have local and general toxic effects. They disrupt absorption in the small intestine, increase the permeability of the intestinal wall, so they cause the penetration of foreign substances into the blood, cause agglutination of erythrocytes. These substances are found in legumes, peanuts, plant germ, fish eggs. Heat treatment destroys lectins.

Cyanogenic amines are found in the kernels, pits of almonds, apricots, and cherries. These kernels contain an enzyme that breaks down these amines. As a result, hydrocyanic acid is formed. This occurs during prolonged storage of sources of cyanogenic amines of nalewka infused on fruits with pips.

Solanine is a toxic compound that forms in greened potato tubers.

Carcinogens are polycyclic aromatic carbohydrates, which are formed in charred parts of foodstuffs, in overheated fats, in smoking products. Carcinogens include nitroso compounds, which are contained in products subjected to salting, smoking, storage in raw, uncut or cooked form at insufficiently low temperature.

Nitroso compounds are also formed in plants grown on soil heavily fertilized with nitrogenous compounds - especially abundant in beets and leafy vegetables.

The role of proteins in the body. Proteins account for about 20% of the dry mass of the cell. Proteins perform plastic and energy functions in the body. 11-13% of the energy consumed by the body comes from proteins. Proteins are not stored in reserves. The biological value of protein is determined by the presence of essential amino acids in it, their ratio with substitutes, digestibility by GI enzymes, the presence of antiprotease fractions (anti-enzymes), antivitamins, allergizing factors in proteins. In this regard, a distinction is made between *complete and incomplete proteins. Complete proteins* contain all essential amino acids (methionine, lysine, tryptophan, phenylalanine, leucine, isoleucine, threonine, valine, and for children - histidine, arginine). In deficient *proteins* there is a deficiency of one or more essential amino acids. The need for amino acids increases in pregnancy, infectious diseases, avitaminosis, and heavy physical activity. A source of complete proteins are milk, dairy products, eggs, meat, fish, liver. A lot of protein in legumes (soybeans, peas, beans). The amino acid composition of proteins from soy, potatoes, rice and rye is close to animal protein. Proteins of animal origin are better digested and assimilated (97%) than vegetable proteins (83-85%). For a more complete utilization of proteins by the organism it is necessary to eliminate antienzyme, antivitamin activity, as well as allergizing effect of proteins - this is achieved by heat treatment. If proteins contain a lot of nucleoproteins (subproducts), nucleic acids are formed in large quantities, which give uric acid, which can lead to gout.

Fats. In normal humans, fat accounts for 10-20%, and in obesity up to 50% of the total mass. Fats perform plastic (for building tissues and synthesizing steroid hormones) and energy function (up to 33% of the energy consumed at the expense of fats). In the body are in two types: structural (protoplasmic) and reserve (depot - in the subcutaneous tissue, in the abdominal cavity - omentum and near the kidneys). Excessive nutrition, hypodynamia, decreased function of the sex glands and thyroid gland cause an increase in fat (excess body weight). The amount of ideal body weight depends on gender, age and height. There are the following ways to determine the proper weight: 1) Broca's index, which is used in some modification: a) for persons with a height of 165 cm and less (P-100), b) for persons with a height of 166-175 cm (P-105), for persons with a height of 176 cm and more (P-110). There is a correction depending on the type of physique: for normostenics (persons with a normal chest) there is no correction, for hyperstenics (persons with a broad chest) 10% is added to the obtained value, for asthenics (persons with a narrow chest) - it is reduced by 10%; 2) in Europe the Kethele index or body mass index (BMI) is widely spread: it is the quotient of the division of body weight (g) by height (cm) squared: BMI = $(B/P)^2$. If the Kethele Index is above 2.4, it indicates that the person has an increased risk of coronary artery disease. Dietary fat comes in animal fat and vegetable fat. Animal fat is mainly represented by triglycerides, which include saturated fatty acids. Fats of plant origin contain mainly unsaturated fatty acids. In the human body, the synthesis of polyunsaturated fatty acids is limited, so these acids (contained in vegetable fat) are essential. These are linoleic acid and arachidonic acid. Fats of vegetable origin are rich in phosphatides (lecithin, kephalin, sphingomyelin), which play an important role in the activity of the body and especially the CNS. With their insufficient intake in the liver is deposited neutral fat, which impairs liver function. Lecithin is important as a regulator of cholesterol metabolism. When the oil is purified (oil refining), these factors are removed. Fat-like substances include sterols - zoosterols and phytosterols - of animal and plant origin, respectively. Phytosterols (beta-sitosterol, ergosterol - vitamin D_2) prevents the absorption of cholesterol in the GI tract. Among zoosterols, cholesterol is an important source of bile acids, steroid hormones. However, excessive utilization of cholesterol causes atherosclerosis. The absorption of liquid fat is much better than solid fat. You should use 80-100 g of fat per day: 25-30 g of vegetable oil, 30-35 g of butter, the rest is cooking fat. Butter has few polyunsaturated fatty acids, but a lot of vitamins such as A, D, E. With insufficient intake of fat in the body, immune properties are reduced, sexual function is impaired, the production of steroid hormones is reduced. If there is insufficient linoleic acid in the diet, there is vascular thrombosis, cancers.

Carbohydrates. The bulk of carbohydrates entering the body are used for energy needs (more than 55% of energy intake). The main source of carbohydrates is plants, which contain up to 80-90% of carbohydrates. These are mainly starch, as well as fiber (ballast substances). Glycogen (of animal origin) in food, as a rule, does not fall into the food, because during the maturation of meat of slaughtered animals, it is destroyed. A daily intake of 400-500 g of carbohydrates is necessary, including at the expense of starch 350-400 g, monosaccharides and disaccharides - 50-100 g, ballast substances - up to 25 g. Excess carbohydrates are transferred to the reserve fat.

Some practical recommendations

Food ration for students (m/w), in g/day: meat and meat products (107/127), fish and fish products (43/53), milk (313/370), cottage cheese (18/21), sour cream (16/18), cheese (16/18), total dairy products (903/1097), eggs (22/26), animal oil (13/16), vegetable oil (22/26), sugar

(80/95), bakery products in terms of flour (343/407), potatoes (268/317), vegetables and melons (317/376), fresh fruits (112/132), dried fruits (4/5).

Features of the food ration for workers of mental labor. For this category of people increased need for proteins and water-soluble vitamins C and B (by 25-30%), vitamin A and beta-carotene. The presence of ballast substances and the use of unrefined food (sugar, oil, bread) is desirable. Energy expenditure is 2400-2800 kcal/day. Energy is formed at the expense of proteins (13%), fats (33%), carbohydrates (54%). The diet should contain proteins of animal origin (not less than 55%), vegetable oil (not less than30%), sugar (not more than 60-70 g / day). A set of the following products is recommended: meat and meat products (200 g), fish (40 g), milk, dairy products (500), cottage cheese (20), sour cream (15), egg (1 pc.), butter (20 g), vegetable oil (20), sugar (70), flour (15), pasta (10), legume cereals (35), potatoes (385), vegetables (300), fruits (200), dried fruits (15).   .

Lecture 24.

**<u>Topic: The functional system that maintains the constancy of
body temperature.</u>**

Objective - to know the main physiological processes that ensure
the maintenance of body temperature constancy: heat production and heat
release, their balance while maintaining isothermia in changing
temperature conditions of the environment; to know the function of
excretory organs, their participation in maintaining homeostasis.

The objectives are.

(a) Give a classification of animals according to the conservation
of body temperature;

b) reveal the role of individual organs in heat production (shivering
and non-shivering thermogenesis);

c) show the ways in which heat is given off and the role of
individual organs in this process;

Content:

A living organism constantly produces heat, which is used to heat
the body. The specific heat capacity of the human body (the amount of
heat required to heat a tissue by 1^0 C) averages 0.83 kcal/kg (1 kcal/kg for
water). It has been found that about 72 kcal/hour is consumed to raise the
body temperature of a person with a mass of 70 kg in resting conditions.
It follows that in the absence of the second process - heat transfer, the
tissues of the organism would be heated hourly by 1.24^0, i.e. overheating
would occur. However, this does not happen due to the functional system
of the organism (FUS), which maintains the constancy of the body
temperature. Let us consider the main links of this system.

The first link of this system, like any other FUS, is the *final useful
adaptive result (FAPR)* - this indicator is the human body temperature. A

52

change in body temperature from the optimal level (increase or decrease) excites the second link - *specific receptors (SR)*. From SRs, impulses through nerve *afferent pathways* (the third link of the FUS) go to the fourth link - the *CNS*. Excitation of this link occurs also by afferent humoral pathway (change of blood temperature directly affects the corresponding CNS structures). Excitation of the corresponding CNS structures causes a flow of efferent impulses to the corresponding working organs - effectors - the fifth link of the FUS.

Changing the work of the corresponding effectors leads to a change in KPPP - the human body temperature. If at maximum change in the work of the effectors (internal reserves of the organism), the body temperature will not be optimal, then the hypothalamus and the cortex of the large hemispheres (HPA) are involved in the excitation process. When the hypothalamus is excited, the endocrine system (ES) becomes involved in the FUS. It should be noted that changes in the function of the ES can be realized due to afferent impulses from the SR. When the PMA is excited, the sixth link of the FUS - *behavior* - begins to function. Now let us consider each link of the FUS separately.

The ultimate beneficial adaptive outcome of this FUS is body temperature. The body temperature of humans and higher animals is maintained at a relatively constant level despite fluctuations in ambient temperature. This constancy of body temperature is called *isothermia*. All animals can be divided into two groups in terms of body temperature constancy:

1) *Poikilothermic* - cold-blooded animals whose body temperature depends mainly on the temperature of the environment: when it decreases, the body temperature also decreases and vice versa. A typical representative of poikilotherms is a frog. In winter, the frog's body temperature approaches zero. In this state, it is still able to make jumps of

no more than 12-15 cm in length. In summer, its body temperature reaches $20\text{-}25^0$, and it can jump up to 1 m;

2) *homoeothermic* - warm-blooded animals that have isothermia or constant body temperature. These animals include mammals. It should be noted that isothermia has a relative character: the temperature of tissues located not deeper than 3 cm from the body surface (skin, subcutaneous tissue, superficial muscles) - the "shell" - largely depends on the external temperature, while the "core" of the body (CNS, internal organs, skeletal muscles located deeper than 3 cm) have a relatively constant temperature regardless of the ambient temperature. Thus, warm-blooded animals have a poikilothermic "shell" and a homoeothermic "core".

Isothermia in the process of ontogenesis develops gradually. In a newborn child, the ability to maintain a constant body temperature is not perfect. As a consequence, cooling (hypothermia) or overheating (hyperthermia) of the body may occur at ambient temperatures that do not affect adults. In them, even a little muscular work (prolonged crying of the baby) can lead to an increase in body temperature. The body of premature babies is even less able to maintain a constant body temperature.

There are microorganisms for which the optimum temperature ranges from 0 to minus 60^0 , e.g. microbes living in the ice. There are also microorganisms that live at temperatures ranging from $+70^0$ to $+120^0$, such as the microbes of hot springs. A number of animals, e.g. bats, rodents, some birds (hummingbirds), belong to the group of *heterothermic* organisms: under some conditions they are poikilothermic and under other conditions they are homoeothermic.

Human body temperature. The temperature of different parts of the "core" is different: in the liver $37.8\text{-}38^0$, in the brain $36.9\text{-}37.8^0$. The temperature of the "core" is best reflected by the temperature of blood in the right heart, where blood from many parts of the body comes. At rest, the blood temperature in the right heart is 36.6-37^0 . In general, the body's "core" temperature is 37^0 .

Human *skin temperature* varies from 24.4^0 to 34^0 . The lowest temperature is in the toes and the highest temperature is in the axilla. The skin of the toes usually has a temperature of 24.4^0 . If a person bathes in cold water, it can drop to 16^0 . To determine the average skin temperature ("envelope"), the temperature is usually measured at 7 standard sites - forehead, foot, shin and thigh, chest, back shoulder, hand. Taking into account the specific gravity of the corresponding surface, the average value is calculated using Wiethe's formula: T = 0.07T foot + 0.32T leg + 0.18T chest + 0.17T back + 0.14T shoulder + 0.05T hand + 0.71T forehead. According to Schmict, the average skin temperature of a naked person at a comfortable temperature is 33-34^0 .

It follows from the above that the concept of "constancy of body temperature" is conditional. Human body temperature is usually judged on the basis of its measurement in the axilla. Here the temperature in a healthy person is equal to 36.5-36.9^0 . In the clinic often (especially in infants) measure the temperature in the rectum, where it is higher than in the axilla, and is equal to a healthy person 37,2-37,5 .^{0}

Body temperature does not remain constant, but fluctuates throughout the day. Circadian, or near-diurnal fluctuations in body temperature are noted - the amplitude of fluctuations reaches 1^0 . Body temperature is minimum in the pre-morning hours (3-4 hours) and maximum in the evening (16-18 hours). In workers working long night shifts, temperature fluctuations can be reversed. Rest and sleep lower and muscle activity raises body temperature.

The phenomenon of axillary temperature asymmetry is known. It occurs in 54% of cases, with a slightly higher temperature in the left axilla than in the right. An increase in asymmetry by 0.5^0 or more indicates pathology.

The skin-temperature coefficient is a temperature gradient that carries useful information for the clinician. This coefficient reflects the difference in skin temperature measured over the iliac (or axillary) artery and the 1st toe of the foot or 1V toe of the hand. In norm it is $3.8\text{-}4^0$ for the upper extremities and 4.9-5.2 for the lower extremities. In case of pathology (in case of deterioration of blood flow of the extremities) it increases.

Specific receptors. These include extra- and interthermo-receptors. Extra-thermo-receptors are located on the skin surface and are represented by cold and heat thermoreceptors. Interoreceptors are located in vessels, internal organs, muscles and the CNS (in the anterior part of the hypothalamus, reticular formation of the brain, spinal cord and cortex of the large hemispheres). Thermoreceptors of the skin are the most fully studied. The most thermoreceptors are on the skin of the head (face) and neck. On average, there is 1 thermoreceptor per 1 mm^2 of skin surface. Cold receptors are located at a depth of 0.17 mm from the skin surface. There are about 250 thousand of them. When they are irritated, the frequency of MFD depends linearly on temperature in the range from 41^0 to 10^0 : the lower the temperature, the higher the pulse frequency. Their optimum sensitivity ranges from 15^0 to 30^0 . Thermal receptors lie deeper - at a distance of 0.3 mm from the skin surface. There are fewer of them - only 30 thousand. They react to temperature changes linearly in the range from 20^0 to 50^0 : the higher the temperature, the higher the frequency of MFD generation. Optimum sensitivity in the range $34\text{-}43^0$. Among cold and heat receptors there are populations with different sensitivities:

1) respond to a temperature change of 0.1^0 (highly sensitive receptors;

2) respond to a temperature change of 1^0 (medium sensitivity receptors);

3) high-threshold, or low sensitivity receptors - react to temperature changes of 10^0. Impulses from skin receptors go to the spinal cord, where second neurons are located, from which the spinothalamic pathway begins and ends in the ventrobasal nuclei of the thalamus. From here, part of the information goes to the sensorimotor zone of the PMA, and part - to the hypothalamic center of thermoregulation. The higher parts of the CNS (PMA and limbic system) provide the formation of heat perception (warm, cold, temperature comfort and discomfort). The hypothalamic region provides regulation of heat production (chemical thermoregulation) and heat dissipation (physical thermoregulation).

Afferent link of FUS consists of: a) nerve pathway, which is represented by spinothalamic pathway; b) humoral pathway - direct action of "hot" or "cold" blood on CNS neurons.

The central link of the FUS. In the central link we can conditionally distinguish: a) the center of thermoregulation in the narrow sense, which is located in the hypothalamus; b) thalamus, hypothalamus (as the highest center of the endocrine and autonomous nervous system; c) PMA.

In the hypothalamus there is a cluster of neurons regulating heat release (heat release department) and heat production (heat production department) The existence of such departments in the hypothalamus was first discovered by C. Bernard. He conducted a "heat shot" (mechanical irritation of the hypothalamus of an animal), after which the body temperature increased. Animals with destroyed nuclei of the preoptic region of the hypothalamus poorly tolerate high ambient temperatures. Irritation of this area with electric current leads to dilation of skin vessels, sweating, and thermal dyspnea. This cluster of nuclei has been called the "center of heat dissipation". When the neurons of the posterior parts of the hypothalamus are destroyed, the animal does not tolerate cold well. Electrical stimulation of this area causes an increase in body temperature, muscle trembling, increased lipolysis, glycogenolysis. The accumulation of these nuclei is called the "heat production center". Destruction of the center of thermoregulation turns a homoeothermic organism into a poikilothermic one. According to K.P. Ivanov (1983, 1984) there are sensory and efferent neurons in the centers of heat production and heat dissipation. Sensory neurons perceive information from thermoreceptors (nerve afferent pathway) and directly from the blood washing the neurons (humoral afferent pathway). If the excitation of the thermoregulation center does not make the body temperature optimal, then the excitation is transmitted to other parts of the hypothalamus and thalamus, which causes the appearance of negative emotions. When negative emotions appear, excitation from the hypothalamus is transmitted to the HPA and the last link of the FUS - behavior - begins to function.

FUS effectors. All FUS effectors can be divided into two groups:

I. Effectors that increase the body's heat output - the work of these organs increases heat output and the body cools down. This mechanism is especially important in maintaining the constancy of body temperature during the stay of the organism in conditions of increased ambient temperature. These organs work by excitation of efferent neurons of the "center of heat dissipation". There are the following ways of heat transfer: a) *heat conduction* - in this case there is a direct transfer of heat by the body in contact with a colder object; b) *convection* - due to the movement and movement of the air heated by heat. At temperature comfort 15% of heat is transferred by this method. The fan increases the heat output by this method; these two methods of heat transfer are realized if the body temperature is below the ambient temperature; c) *heat* radiation, due to the emission of infrared rays - this method is realized if the body temperature is below and equal to the ambient temperature. In conditions of comfort temperature, up to 60% of heat is carried out due to this mechanism; it should be noted that in all the above mentioned ways of heat transfer a significant role is played by skin blood flow: when its intensity increases due to a decrease in the tone of smooth muscle cells of arterioles and closure of arteriovenous shunts - heat transfer increases significantly. This is also promoted by an increase in the volume of circulating blood; d) *evaporation of water* - this method is carried out when the ambient temperature rises above body temperature. In this case, the heat transfer occurs at the expense of energy expenditure (evaporation of 1 ml of water is accompanied by energy expenditure of 0.58 kcal). There are two types of evaporation, or perspiration: non-sensible and sensible perspiration. Insensible perspiration is the evaporation of water from the mucous membranes of the respiratory tract and water that seeps through the epithelium of the skin. In a day, up to 400 ml of water evaporates through the respiratory tract (232 kcal of heat is given off). When the temperature rises, this value increases (thermal dyspnea). On average, about 240 ml of water seeps through the epidermis per day. This value does not depend on environmental factors. Both types of perspiration in a day allow 371 kcal to be given up. Perceptible perspiration, or the release of heat by evaporation of sweat. At a comfortable temperature, an average of 400-500 ml of sweat is secreted per day, hence up to 300 kcal is given off. If necessary, sweating can increase up to 12 liters per day (gives off heat up to 7000 kcal). In an hour sweat glands can produce up to 1.5 liters, and according to some sources up to 3 liters. By chemical composition sweat is a hypotonic solution (0.3% sodium chloride, urea, glucose, amino acids, ammonium, small amounts of lactic acid), pH ranges from 4.2-7, on average pH = 6. Spinal cord neurons involved in the regulation of sweating are located in T_2 -L_2 . There are three types of sweating disorders: 1) anhidrosis - complete absence of sweating; 2) hypohidrosis - partial reduction of sweating; 3) hyperhidrosis - excessive sweat production.

The contribution of each mode of heat transfer in the body is different. Under conditions of thermal comfort, the bulk of heat is given off by conduction, convection and radiation, and only 19-20% by evaporation. At high ambient temperatures - up to 75-90% of heat is given off by evaporation. There are two heat flows in the body: 1) internal flow - heat transfer from internal organs to the skin. In this significant role is given to the blood - a kind of "heat pipe" of the body; 2) external flow - heat transfer from the skin to the external environment. When considering the mechanism of heat transfer, usually mean this flow. The organs of heat transfer include: 1) *skin* (82% of heat is given off through the skin). Heat transfer through the skin is realized by two mechanisms: a) due to vascular reactions - expansion of skin vessels. In this case, heat transfer occurs in three ways: heat conduction, convection, heat radiation; b) through sweating, in this case, heat transfer occurs by evaporation; 2) *lungs* (13%) through the lungs heat transfer is carried out by evaporation of water vapor saturating exhaled air. At high ambient temperature, the respiratory center is reflexively excited, at low temperature - depressed, breathing becomes less deep. 3) *gastrointestinal tract* (4%) - to warm food, by heat conduction; 4) *heating of feces and urine* (1%).

Physical thermoregulation includes *changes in body position.* When a dog or cat is cold, they curl up in a ball, thereby reducing the heat transfer surface; when it is hot, they adopt a position in which the heat transfer surface is maximized. This is also true for humans, who "curl up in a ball" when sleeping in a cold room.

Rudimentary significance for humans is the *manifestation of the reaction of skin muscles ("gooseflesh").* In animals, this changes the cellularity of the wool cover and improves the insulating role of wool.

II. Effectors contributing to heat-production. The work of these organs increases the formation of heat in the body - there is an increase in temperature. This mechanism is of great importance when the ambient temperature decreases. Enhancement of functions of these organs is carried out due to excitation of efferent neurons of the center of heat production. In this case, the release of energy in the body is carried out due to the oxidation of nutrients (proteins, fats and carbohydrates). The importance of organs and tissues in heat generation is different: 1) *skeletal muscles* (60% of heat in the body is generated by muscle contraction). There is an involuntary contraction of muscles - *shivering*. Heat generated by involuntary muscle contraction is called shivering *thermogenesis*. In this case, metabolic processes in the body are significantly increased, the consumption of oxygen and carbohydrates by muscle tissue increases, which entails an increase in heat generation. Even arbitrary imitation of shivering increases heat generation by 200%. If myorelaxants - substances that disrupt the transmission of excitation from nerve to muscle and thereby eliminate shivering - are introduced into the body, the body temperature drops much faster. Skeletal muscles also contract due to impulses from the PMA - this is an *arbitrary contraction*. The aggregate of arbitrary contractions of skeletal muscles constitute a particular *behavior*. It should be noted that when the body is horizontal (lying down), but with tense muscles, there is an increase in heat generation (due to the intensity of oxidative processes) by 10%. Small motor activity leads to an increase in heat generation by 50-80%, and heavy muscle load - by 400-500%. During muscle contraction, ATP hydrolysis increases and the flow of secondary heat increases, which is used to warm the organism. When the temperature of the environment and blood decreases, the first reaction of muscles is an increase in thermoregulatory tone (microvibrations). On average, when it appears, heat production increases by 20-45% of the initial level. With more significant cooling, thermoregulatory tone turns into muscle cold shivering. Shivering is an involuntary rhythmic activity of superficially located muscles, as a result of which heat production increases 2-3 times. At first, tremor occurs in the muscles of the head and neck, then the trunk and then the extremities. In this case, signals from hypothalamic neurons go through the red nucleus ("central tremor pathway") to the alpha-motoneurons of the spinal cord, from where the signal goes to the corresponding muscles, causing their activity. In skeletal muscles, heat production can occur through non-contractile thermogenesis - by reducing the efficiency of oxidative phosphorylation; 2) *liver (30%)*. In the liver, thermogenesis occurs mainly due to activation of glycogenolysis and subsequent glucose oxidation. The temperature of hepatic vein blood is higher than the temperature of arterial blood, indicating the intensity of heat generation in this organ. Due to intensive oxidation processes in the liver, this organ is called the "biochemical kitchen" of our body; 3) *brown fat* takes a special place in the heat formation of the body, especially in newborns and inhabitants of the Arctic zones who have a significant amount of it. Brown color of fat is given by a greater number of sympathetic nerve fiber endings and a greater number of mitochondria. Brown fat increases heat production due to lipolysis under the influence of sympathetic influences and adrenaline. Brown fat is located in the occipital region, between the shoulder blades, in the mediastinum along the course of large vessels, in the axillae. Due to the high rate of oxidation of fatty acids in brown adipose tissue, the process of heat generation is much faster than in normal. The heat generated due to non-scratic thermogenesis in muscles, glycogenolysis in the liver and lipolysis in brown fat is called non-fatty *thermogenesis;* 4) *other organs* (10%) - due to oxidative processes in all other organs and tissues of the body. Regulation of non-fat thermogenesis is realized by activation of the sympathetic system and production of hormones of the thyroid gland and the brain layer of the adrenal glands. Heat generation in the body is carried out due to oxidation of proteins, fats and carbohydrates in the body. In humans, increased heat generation (by increasing the intensity of metabolism) is noted when the ambient temperature becomes lower than the *optimal* temperature (comfort zone). For a person in ordinary light clothing, this zone is within $+18+20^0$, and for the naked is equal to $+28^0$. The optimal temperature while in the water is higher than in the air. This is due to the fact that water, which has a high heat capacity and thermal conductivity, cools the body 14 times stronger than air. In this regard, in a cool bath, metabolism increases much more than when staying in the air at the same temperature.

The endocrine system is also one of the effectors involved in body temperature change. When the heat production center is irritated (when the ambient temperature increases), thyreoliberin production in the hypothalamus is inhibited, which leads to a decrease in thyroid function. When the center of heat production is irritated (when the ambient temperature decreases), thyreoliberin production increases, which leads to an increase in thyroid function. Of the glands of internal secretion in the regulation of body temperature are involved, mainly thyroid and adrenal glands. With the participation of the thyroid gland in the blood are released hormones (thyroxine and triiodothyrosine) that increase the intensity of metabolism, increasing heat production. The adrenal glands are involved in the release of adrenaline into the blood, which: 1) increases oxidative processes in the muscles and increases heat generation; 2) narrows skin vessels, reducing heat production.

Thus, when the heat production center is excited, there is: 1) excitation of spinal cord motoneurons and contraction of skeletal muscles (shivering thermogenesis); 2) excitation of spinal cord sympathetic neurons, which leads to glycogenolysis in skeletal muscles and liver, as well as to lipolysis of brown fat (non-shivering thermogenesis). When the center of heat production is excited, the following occurs: 1) excitation of sympathetic neurons of the spinal cord with increased work of sweat glands; with increased sweat production, kallikrein activity increases, which leads to an increase in the concentration of bradykinin in the blood. Bradykinin promotes sweating and dilation of skin vessels; 2) excitation of the depressor section of the vasomotor center with decreased activity of spinal cord neurons, which leads to vasodilation and increased heat production.

Behavior is an external link of the FUS. This link of the FUS begins to function when the internal reserve of the organism is exhausted. If at maximum function of all effectors involved in temperature regulation (at increasing ambient temperature - participation of organs that increase heat release; at decreasing ambient temperature - participation of organs that increase heat production), the body temperature will not be optimal, then excitation from the hypothalamus passes to the PMA - *behavior* occurs, which contributes to the change of body temperature to the optimal value.

HYPOTHERMIA AND HYPERTHERMIA

Hypothermia is a condition in which the body temperature is below 35^0 C. Hypothermia occurs most quickly when immersed in cold water. In recent years, artificial hypothermia is used in surgical practice during heart and CNS surgeries. In this case, the temperature is reduced to $24\text{-}28^0$ C. The meaning of hypothermia is that it sharply reduces the metabolism of the body due to the shift of the dissociation curve of oxyhemoglobin to the left decreases the body's need for oxygen. As a result, longer exsanguination of the brain becomes tolerable (instead of 3-5 min at normal temperature up to 15-20 min at a temperature of $24\text{-}28^0$) and patients more easily tolerate temporary shutdown of the heart and respiratory arrest. When using hypothermia it is necessary to exclude adaptive reactions of the organism (work of separate links of FUS). For this purpose, drugs that turn off impulse transmission in ANS (ganglioblockers) and stop impulse transmission from nerves to skeletal muscles (myorelaxants) are used.

At short-term and not excessively intensive effects of cold on the body changes in the thermal balance and lowering the temperature of the internal environment does not occur. At the same time, it contributes to the development of colds and exacerbation of chronic inflammatory processes. In this regard is of great importance *hardening* of the *body*. Hardening is achieved by repeated exposure to low temperatures of increasing intensity. In weak people hardening should begin with water procedures of neutral temperature (32^0 C) and lower the temperature by 1^0 C every 2-3 days. The effect of hardening is manifested not only in water procedures, but also when exposed to cold air. In this case, hardening occurs faster if the impact of cold is combined with active muscle activity.

Hyperthermia - a condition in which the body temperature rises above 37^0 C. It occurs with prolonged action of high ambient temperature, especially in humid air (in this case, the body's heat transfer by means of evaporation is sharply impaired). Hyperthermia may also occur under the influence of some endogenous factors that increase heat generation in the body (thyroxine, adrenaline, fatty acids, etc.). Sharp hyperthermia (increase in body temperature up to 40-41^0) is accompanied by a severe general condition of the body and is called *heat stroke.*

Hyperthermia should be distinguished from a rise in temperature under unchanged external conditions. In this case, there is a disruption of thermoregulation in the body. An example of such a violation is infectious fever. One of the reasons for its occurrence is the high sensitivity of hypothalamic centers to bacterial toxins. The introduction of a minimal amount of bacterial toxin into the anterior hypothalamus is accompanied by a temperature rise for many hours.

Lecture 25.

Topic: Excretory organs (kidney, lungs, skin, digestive tract and mammary glands), their participation in maintaining homeostasis of the internal environment.

Objective - to know the function of excretory organs, their participation in the maintenance of homeostasis.

The objectives are.

(a) Point out the excretory function of the lungs, skin, digestive tract;

b) reveal the elements cf the nephron as a morphofunctional unit of the kidneys;

c) show the processes occurring in the nephron (filtration, secretion, reabsorption, incretion) and their mechanisms;

d) provide an understanding of non-sugar diabetes.

Content:

Excretion is the process of freeing the body from metabolic products that cannot be used by the body, foreign and toxic substances, excess water, salts, and organic compounds. The organs of excretion include the *kidneys, lungs, skin (sweat and sebaceous glands), digestive tract, and mammary glands*. Of these organs, the mammary and sebaceous glands are special excretory organs because they secrete substances that are beneficial to the body. The products of sebaceous and mammary glands - sebum and *milk* have an independent physiological significance - milk as a food product for newborns, and sebum to lubricate the skin. The main importance of excretory organs is to maintain the constancy of the composition and volume of fluids of the internal environment of the body, primarily blood.

The lungs remove from the body: 1) CO_2 and thus participates in maintaining the constancy of blood pH (when the pH decreases, the release of CO_2 increases, and when the pH increases, the release of CO_2 decreases). Hypoventilation contributes to respiratory (gas) acidosis, and hyperventilation - to the emergence of respiratory alkalosis; 2) water and thus participates in the maintenance of body temperature by evaporation of heat; 3) toxic substances (excess of narcotic substances and alcohol vapors).

Salivary and gastric glands excrete: 1) heavy metals; 2) a number of drugs (morphine, quinine, salicylates); 3) foreign organic compounds.

The liver removes a number of products of nitrogenous metabolism, excess bile pigments and acids from the blood with bile.

The pancreas and intestinal glands eliminate heavy metals and drugs.

The glands of the skin due to *sweat* glands secrete: 1) water (its evaporation from the skin surface helps maintain body temperature); 2) some organic substances, particularly urea; 3) lactic acid, especially during strenuous muscular work. *Sebaceous* glands secrete *sebum* to lubricate the skin.

The mammary glands secrete breast milk as food for newborns.

Kidney Function. The kidneys are the main excretory organs. The main functions of the kidneys:

1) are involved in the regulation of the volume of blood and other body fluids, ionic composition of internal fluids, acid-base balance, blood pressure and erythropoiesis;

2) They participate in the excretion of end products of nitrogen metabolism and excess organic substances from food or formed during metabolism;

3) are involved in the secretion of enzymes and physiologically active substances (hemopoietins, renin, bradykinin, prostaglandins, vitamin D).[3]

The structural and functional unit of the kidney is the nephron, which consists of the following elements:

1) bringing arteriole;

2) The nephron tubule (primary capillary network);

3) the exporting arteriole;

4) secondary capillary network;

5) venule; 6) Baumann-Schumlansky capsule cavity;

7) The first-order tortuous tubule, or proximal tortuous tubule;

8) straight downward channel;

9) loop of Henle;

10) ascending rectal tubule;

11) The second-order tortuous tubule, or distal tortuous tubule;

12) collecting tube.

The following processes occur in the nephron: 1) filtration; 2) reabsorption; 3) secretion; and 4) incretion. The first three processes ensure *urine formation.*

Clot filtration - penetration of water and low molecular weight compounds from the tubules into the capsular cavity. There are three barriers to filtration: the endothelium of the tubular capillary, the basal membrane and the inner leaflet of the capsule. The force favoring filtration is the *hydrostatic pressure of blood* (70 mmHg) in the capillaries of the tubule. The forces preventing filtration include: *oncotic pressure of blood* (30 mmHg) and *hydrostatic pressure of ultrafiltrate* in the Bowman-Shumlansky capsule (20 mmHg). The *effective filtration pressure*, on which the rate of glomerular filtration depends, is determined by the difference between the pressure promoting filtration and the pressure preventing it (70-30-20=20 mmHg). The amount of ultrafiltrate (*primary urine*) reaches 150-180 liters per day. The filtrate rate reaches 120 ml/min in men and 110 ml/min in women.

Canalicular reabsorption is the back absorption of water and some substances necessary for the body from primary urine into the blood. From 150-180 liters of primary urine due to reabsorption is formed only 1.5-2 liters of final, or secondary, urine. Reabsorption of substances in different parts of the nephron is not the same. In the proximal segment of the nephron from the ultrafiltrate completely reabsorbed glucose, amino acids, vitamins, proteins, trace elements. In subsequent sections of the nephron, only ions and water are reabsorbed. Reabsorption is influenced by the following factors: 1) the concentration of *threshold and non-threshold* substances. Threshold *substances are those* that are reabsorbed. The reabsorption of these substances depends on their concentration in the blood. For these substances there are threshold concentrations in the blood - their minimum concentration in the blood, when these substances are not completely reabsorbed. For example, glucose is completely reabsorbed when its blood concentration is equal to or less than 10 mmol/L. When the blood glucose concentration increases beyond this value, some glucose is excreted in the urine, resulting in glucosuria - the appearance of glucose in the final urine. *Threshold-free substances* - do not undergo reabsorption (they are completely excreted by urine), so there is no threshold concentration in the blood for them. For example, the polysaccharide inulin and sulfates. If these substances have entered the ultrafiltrate, they are not reabsorbed. It follows from the above that increasing the concentration of threshold substances in the blood above a threshold value decreases their reabsorption, and this leads to a decrease in water reabsorption. An increase in threshold-free substances in the ultrafiltrate contributes to a decrease in water reabsorption; 2) the *rotary-*

countercurrent system (this system combines descending and ascending straight tubules, as well as the loop of Henle). This system is of great importance in the reabsorption of sodium ions and water. The epithelium of the ascending straight tubule has the ability to actively transport sodium ions into the intercellular fluid and is almost impermeable to water. In contrast, the epithelium of the descending direct tubule is permeable to water but lacks mechanisms for active transport of sodium ions. The ultrafiltrate, passing through the descending tubule, gives up water and thus becomes more concentrated. At the same time, water reabsorption occurs passively due to the fact that in the ascending section there is active reabsorption of sodium ions, which increase the osmotic pressure of intercellular fluid and thus contribute to the reabsorption of water from the descending direct tubule. In turn, reabsorption of water leads to an increase in urine concentration in the nephron loop, which facilitates the transfer of sodium ions into the intercellular fluid; 3) *hormones* - vasopressin (anti-diuretic hormone - ADH) and aldosterone. ADH is a hormone that is formed in the hypothalamus and accumulates in the posterior lobe of the pituitary gland. Once in the bloodstream, this hormone affects the collecting tube of the nephron and increases the activity of the enzyme hyaluronidase, which promotes the breakdown of hyaluronic acid and increases the porosity of the wall. These changes result in increased water reabsorption. In the absence of ADH or a small amount of ADH (nonsugar diabetes), water reabsorption in the collecting tube is impaired and the amount of end urine increases (polyuria). When ADH is increased, conversely, water reabsorption in the collecting tube is increased, decreased (oliguria) or absent (anuria). Aldosterone is a hormone of the adrenal cortex (mineralocorticoid). This hormone mainly affects the ascending rectal tubule and increases sodium reabsorption, which in turn, through the pivot-optic system, increases water reabsorption. Insulin affects glucose and water reabsorption indirectly (through regulation of glucose concentration). When insulin secretion is insufficient (diabetes mellitus), the amount of glucose in the blood increases. If the glucose concentration reaches a threshold value, its reabsorption in the tubules decreases, which leads to a decrease in water reabsorption.

Canalicular secretion in which the epithelial cells of the nephron capture some substances from the blood and interstitial fluid and carries them into the lumen of the tubules. The secretion allows rapid excretion of organic acids, bases, and ions. Another variant of tubule secretion is the release into the lumen of the tubules of new substances synthesized in the cells of the nephron. Thus, in the cells of renal tubules ammonia is synthesized in the deamination of amino acids from amino groups (amoniogenesis), which captures hydrogen ions from the blood, turning into ammonium and is excreted into the tubule cavity. This is one of the mechanisms by which blood pH is maintained by the kidneys. Hypuric acid is also synthesized from benzoic acid and glycocol in renal tubule cells.

The kidneys produce a number of physiologically active substances that are excreted into the blood. The implementation of the incretory function is associated with the juxtaglomerular apparatus, which is located at the entrance to the tubule between the supplying and exporting arterioles of the tubule and part of the wall of the distal tubule. It includes granular cells of the supply arteriole, cells of the dense patch of the distal tubule and special cells that contact both groups of cells.

The kidneys produce the following physiologically active substances:

1) *renin* - formed by granular cells and is a proteolytic enzyme that facilitates the cleavage of the inactive peptide angiotensin I from

angiotensinogen. Two amino acids are cleaved from angiotensin I and it is converted into the active vasoconstrictor, angiotensin II. In addition, angiotensin II affects the rate of reabsorption of sodium ions, stimulates the secretion of aldosterone by cells of the adrenal cortex. The homeostatic value of renin is that it decreases glomerular filtration and leads to the preservation of the volume of extracellular fluid and blood and prevents the loss of sodium ions;

2) *vitamin* D_3 - kidney cells extract a prohormone from blood plasma formed in the liver - vitamin D_3 and convert it into physiologically active hormone D_3 . This hormone stimulates the formation of calcium-binding protein in intestinal cells, which is necessary for the absorption of calcium ions, it promotes the release of calcium from bones and regulates its reabsorption in the renal tubules;

3) Hemopoietins *(erythro-, leuko-, and thrombopoietins),* which are involved in hematopoiesis;

4) *kinins*, which are strong vasodilators involved in the regulation of renal blood flow and sodium excretion;

5) *prostaglandins*, including *prostaglandin A_3 (medullin),* which is formed in the renal medulla and increases renal blood flow and sodium ion excretion without altering glomerular filtration. Medullin decreases the sensitivity of tubule cells to ADH;

6) *plasminogen activator (urokinase),* which activates plasminogen, converting it into plasmin (fibrinolysin) and prevents blood clotting. It has been found that the fibrinolytic activity of blood taken in the renal vein is significantly higher than in the renal artery.

Metabolic function of the kidneys - provides maintenance of a constant level of proteins, carbohydrates and lipids in the fluids of the internal environment. Albumin and globulins do not pass through the membrane of the tubule, but low molecular weight proteins, peptides are freely filtered. Consequently, the tubule cavity constantly receives hormones, altered proteins. Cells of the proximal tubule capture them and break them down to amino acids, which are transported through the basal plasma membrane into the extracellular fluid and then into the blood. This helps to restore the body's amino acid pool.

The kidneys have an active glucose formation system. During prolonged fasting, almost half of the total amount of glucose entering the blood is synthesized in the kidneys. The kidneys use organic acids to synthesize glucose and thereby help stabilize blood pH, so in alkalosis, glucose synthesis from acidic substrates is reduced.

Renal involvement in lipid metabolism is due to the fact that the kidney extracts free fatty acids from the blood and their oxidation is largely responsible for kidney function. These acids are bound to albumin in the plasma and therefore they are not filtered. They enter the cells of the nephron from the intercellular fluid. Free fatty acids are incorporated into phospholipids, triacylglycerides and as these compounds enter the blood.

The role of the kidneys in the regulation of blood osmotic pressure. In normal humans, the osmotic pressure (osmolarity) of blood is within 290 mosmol/kg of water. Osmoreceptors are localized in the area of the supraoptic nucleus of the hypothalamus, in the liver, heart, kidneys and other organs. According to Vernay's osmoreceptor hypothesis, when blood osmotic pressure increases, the flow of impulses from osmoreceptors increases, which leads to the release of ADH from the neurohypophysis, water reabsorption in the collecting tubes of the nephron increases, and blood osmotic pressure decreases. ADH production increases under the influence of painful stimulation - painful anuria occurs.

The role of the kidneys in the regulation of circulating blood volume. Volumoreceptors (stretch receptors), which are localized in the arterial and venous systems - in the zones of low and high pressure, play a role in the regulation of the volume of circulating blood and interstitial fluid. There are volumoreceptors in the wall of the left atrium. With increasing blood flow through the pulmonary veins, the wall of the left atrium stretches, exciting volumoreceptors, there is a flow of afferent impulses. These impulses increase vagus tone, which leads to negative effects on the heart and decreased blood flow in the small circle of circulation. At the same time these impulses arrive in the supraoptic nucleus of hypothalamus - ADH secretion decreases, water reabsorption in the collecting tubes of nephron decreases, diuresis (polyuria) increases, which leads to normalization of CCA. Part of volumoreceptors is located in the carotid sinus and in the region of the aortic arch. When blood pressure decreases, ADH secretion increases and CCA increases. CABG is also regulated by the renin-angiotensin-aldosterone system. When CCA decreases, blood pressure decreases, which leads to increased production of renin, angiotensin II is formed, which increases aldosterone production. This causes an increase in sodium reabsorption, followed by water reabsorption. As a result, the ODC increases.

The role of kidneys in the regulation of blood ionic composition. Kidneys play a major role in maintaining the concentration of sodium, potassium, calcium and chlorine ions in the blood: 1) *sodium ions* - their concentration in the blood is maintained at the level of 140-143 mmol/L. When the level of sodium in the blood decreases, the production of aldosterone increases (including by increasing the renin-angiotensin-aldosterone system), which increases the activity of the sodium-potassium pump in the renal tubules and promotes increased reabsorption of sodium. With excessive sodium ions in the blood, the production of sodium uretic hormone (atriopeptin), which is produced in the hypothalamus and reduces sodium reabsorption, increases. It should be noted that the level of ADH indirectly affects the concentration of sodium ions in the blood: an increase in ADH increases water reabsorption and thereby reduces the concentration of sodium ions; 2) *potassium ions* - their concentration in the blood is kept at 4.5 mmol/L. The level of potassium in the blood is maintained by secretion: when potassium in the blood increases above normal, its secretion increases, this is due to the influence of aldosterone (activates the sodium-potassium pump, increasing sodium reabsorption and potassium secretion. Insulin decreases potassium secretion. In acidosis, potassium secretion decreases (sodium is exchanged for hydrogen, so potassium is not secreted), and in alkalosis increases; 3) *calcium ions* - their concentration is maintained at 2.5 mmol/L. Paratgormone increases calcium reabsorption, and thyrocalcitonin decreases. Signals to the appropriate glands come from calcium receptors located in the liver; 4) chlorine *anions* - their concentration is within 100 mmol/L. Usually reabsorption of chlorine occurs behind sodium ions, so when sodium reabsorption increases, chlorine reabsorption also increases.

The role of the kidneys in the regulation of acid-base equilibrium (pH). Maintenance of blood pH by the kidneys is realized by the following mechanisms: 1) by regulation of sodium bicarbonate reabsorption. In acidosis, the efficiency of bicarbonate reabsorption increases, while in alkalosis it decreases. In acidosis, excess hydrogen ions are taken up by the epithelial cells of the tubule and secreted into the tubule lumen, which displaces the sodium ion from bicarbonate, converting it to carbonic acid. Under the influence of carboanhydrase (localized on the apical part of the epithelial cell), carbonic acid is broken down into water and carbon dioxide. Carbon dioxide enters the cell, where it is converted into carbonic acid under the influence of carboanhydrase. It dissociates into hydrogen ion and HCO anion$_3$. The hydrogen ion leaves the cell into the lumen of the tubule and displaces the sodium from the bicarbonate again. Thus the secretion of hydrogen in exchange for sodium eventually results in all bicarbonate passing from the primary urine into the blood and the excess hydrogen ions escaping into the urine; 2) excretion of hydrogen ions by phosphate buffer. Hydrogen ions secreted into the tubule lumen bind to phosphate ($Na_2 HPO_4$) and displace sodium from it, becoming $NaH_2 PO_4$, which leaves the kidney and carries away excess hydrogen ions; 3) through the process of *ammoniogenesis* - when urine pH drops to 5 or less, the phosphate buffer is depleted and ammonia synthesis begins in the tubule cells as a result of deamination of amino acids (glutamic acid). Ammonia captures hydrogen ion from the blood and is converted to ammonium, which is secreted into the tubule cavity where it displaces sodium from sodium chloride. This produces $NH_4 Cl$, which is excreted with the urine. The released sodium is reabsorbed into the blood and combines with the anion HCO_3 , replenishing the capacity of the bicarbonate buffer.

Regulation of kidney function. There are two main mechanisms of kidney function regulation: 1) *nerve regulation* - irritation of sympathetic fibers innervating kidneys leads to constriction of blood vessels in kidneys. Narrowing of the supply arterioles leads to a decrease in filtration due to a decrease in hydrostatic pressure in the tubules. Constriction of the outflow arterioles increases filtration by increasing the pressure in the tubules. Sympathetic influences stimulate sodium reabsorption. Parasympathetic influences activate reabsorption of glucose and secretion of organic acids. With painful stimuli, there may be a decrease in urine output up to complete cessation (*painful anuria*). The mechanism of painful anuria is as follows: a) there is a spasm of supplying arterioles with increased activity of the sympathetic nervous system and secretion of catecholamines by the adrenal glands, this leads to a sharp decrease in filtration; b) pain activates the hypothalamic nuclei, increases ADH secretion, increases water reabsorption, decreases diuresis, up to its disappearance; 2) *conditionally-reflex change in* diuresis. Anuria, coming under painful irritation, as well as an increase in diuresis can be reproduced conditionally-reflexively. Repeated introduction of water into the dog's body in combination with the action of a conditioned stimulus leads to the formation of a conditioned reflex accompanied by an increase in urine output. Conditioned reflex change of diuresis testifies to participation in regulation of kidney work of the higher parts of CNS - cortex of large hemispheres; 3) *humoral regulation of* kidney activity plays the leading role. Kidney function is influenced by a number of hormones: ADH, aldosterone, parathormone, thyroxine, thyrocalcitonin. The mechanism of their action has been described above.

Lecture 26.

Topic: General questions of physiology of the endocrine system.

The aim is to know the basic mechanisms of hormone action, self-regulation of the endocrine system, functional relationships of the glands of internal secretion and the nervous system, hypothalamic neurosecretes and, corresponding to them, tropic hormones.

The objectives are.

(a) Give a physiological classification of hormones;

b) reveal the mechanisms of action of hormones (extracellular and intracellular);

c) Show on Functional links between the hypothalamus and pituitary gland (liberins, statins and tropic hormones);

d) indicate the regulation of hormone release into the blood.

Content:

Endocrinology is a science that studies the development, structure and function of the glands of internal secretion and hormone-producing cells, biosynthesis, mechanism of action and features of hormones, their secretion in norm and pathology, as well as diseases resulting from impaired hormone production.

Internal secretion glands, or endocrine glands, produce hormone. Unlike the external secretion glands, or exocrine glands, these glands have no ducts and secrete their secretions directly into the blood, lymph and other tissue fluids. Hence their name - endocrine (from Greek endon - inside, krinein - to secrete). The term "internal secretion" was introduced by the famous French physiologist Claude Bernard in 1855. C. Bernard considered all organs to be glands with internal secretion in a broad sense, since they secrete the products of their metabolism into the blood.

The year 1849 is considered to be the birth year of endocrinology. In this year, Adolf Berthold established the fact that the effects of castration in a capon were eliminated after transplanting rooster testes into its abdomen. For the first time it was shown experimentally that substances from certain organs have a regulating effect on metabolism and determine the development of secondary sexual characteristics. By this time there are descriptions of specific diseases of endocrine glands: thyroid gland - Graves in 1835, Bazedovoy in 1840; adrenal glands - Addison in 1855. In 1889 Broun-Sekar reported on experiments conducted on himself - extracts from the testes of animals had a "rejuvenating" effect on the aging body of the scientist (he was 72 years old). In 1889-1890 Mering and Minkowski established the connection between diabetes mellitus and the violation of the pancreas, and in 1901 L.V. Sobolev showed the endocrine function of the islets of Langerhans, which was identified in 1921 by F. Bunting and C. Best as insulin. In 1905, British physiologists Baylis and Starling introduced the term "hormone" (from Greek Hormo - prompting, excitement). They isolated secretin from the wall of the 12th intestine, which causes an increase in pancreatic secretion. Currently, endocrinology continues to develop intensively.

It becomes obvious that the production of physiologically active substances is not only due to the function of internal secretion glands, but also many non-endocrine organs: gastrointestinal tract, kidneys, liver, heart produce hormones and hormonoids. At the end of the last century, chromaffin cells were discovered in the intestine, which were intensely stained with chromium. Subsequently, similar cells were identified in the esophagus, bronchi, and other parts of the respiratory system. The Austrian pathologist Feirter, who discovered these cells, grouped them into a paracrine system, believing that they produce substances similar to hormones. English histologist Pearce in the 50-ies of the twentieth century found that all these cells are able to absorb amino acids (precursors of hormones) introduced from outside and break them down by decarboxylation, and from their residues to synthesize hormones. He called this process "Amine Precursor Aptake and Decarboxylation." The first letters of four of these words formed the acronym, APUD (1968). The cells were named "apudocytes". Now more than 50 types of apudocytes are known, synthesizing more than 30 hormones, including serotonin, melatonin, adrenaline, histamine, insulin, gastrin, secretin, pancreosimine, bombesin, enkephalins, endorphins and others. The APUD system is given much attention due to the fact that without apudocytes the normal vital activity of the organism is disturbed.

The number of hormones being discovered is increasing. However, one should be wary of classifying a newly discovered biologically active substance as a hormone without sufficient evidence. Classical endocrinology requires the following evidence to establish its hormonal activity:

1) the presence of distinct manifestations of a "dropout" hormonal effect that occurs after removal of the hormone-secreting organ;

2) elimination of the phenomena of "loss" in the application of substitution therapy (auto- or homotransplants, extracts from the organ in question);

3) the purified preparation obtained from this organ (or synthesized) must have a qualitatively specific hormonal action.

All hormones are organic compounds. According to their chemical structure, they can be divided into two main groups: 1) hormones that are amino acids and their derivatives - polypeptides and proteins; 2) steroidal, or lipid, hormones. The first group includes: a) hormones represented by complex proteins (glucoproteins) - thyroid, follicle-stimulating, luteinizing; b) peptide hormones consisting of 30-90 amino acid residues

- adrenocorticotropic hormone, somatotropic, melanocytostimulating, prolactin, paratgormone, insulin, glucagon; c) oligopeptides consisting of a small number of amino acid residues - liberins, statins, oxytacin, gastrointestinal hormones.

Steroid hormones are derivatives of cholesterol: cholesterol is converted to pregnenalone, from which all major steroid hormones originate - corticosterone, cortisol, aldosterone, estradiol, progestins, estriol, estrone, testosterone. In addition, this group includes arachidonic acid and its derivatives - prostaglandins, prostacyclins, thromboxanes, leukotrienes. From the position of permeability, it should be noted that of the hormones derived from amino acids, only thyroid hormones are able to pass through cell membranes.

Hormones can be divided into three groups according to their functionality (physiological classification): I) effector hormones - these hormones are formed in peripheral glands of internal secretion (thyroid, parathyroid, pancreas, placenta, ovaries, testes, adrenal glands) and influence directly on organs and tissues (target object); II) tropic hormones - formed in the anterior lobe of the pituitary gland and influence peripheral glands of internal secretion. The following main tropic hormones are distinguished: (a) thyroid hormone (TTH) - affects the thyroid gland and enhances its function; (b) somatotropic hormone (STH) - affects the liver, where in response somatomedins are synthesized, which influence the growth of organs and tissues; (c) adrenocorticotropic hormone (ACTH) - affects the cortical layer of the adrenal glands and enhances the production of corticosteroids; (d) gonadotropic hormone (GTH). These include: 1) follicle-stimulating hormone (FSH) - affects the ovaries (promotes follicle maturation) in women and the testes (promotes sperm maturation) in men; 2) luteinizing hormone (LH) - promotes the development of the corpus luteum; e) luteotropic hormone (LTH), or prolactin - affects the mammary glands and increases milk production; III) liberins (releasing hormones) and statins (inhibitor hormones) - are formed in the hypothalamus and act on the anterior lobe of the pituitary gland, stimulating (liberins) or inhibiting (statins) the production of the corresponding tropic hormones. There are the following types of liberins: 1) thyreoliberin - increases the production of TTH; 2) corticoliberin - increases the production of ACTH; 3) foliberin - increases the production of FSH; 4) luliberin - increases the production of LH; 5) prolactoliberin - increases the production of LTG; 6) somatoliberin - increases the production of STH. The following statins are distinguished: 1) somatostatin - inhibits STH production; 2) prolactostatin - inhibits LTH production.

Hormone receptors. Currently, 60 hormone receptors have been identified, of which 50% are localized on the membranes of the target cell, and in the remaining cases inside the cell. Hormones that are unable to penetrate the plasma membrane have receptors on the cell surface. Intracellular receptors are used to sense steroid hormones such as glucocorticoids, mineralocorticoids, estrogens, androgens, progestins, and thyroid hormones (thyroxine, triiodothyronine). Receptors for many hormones have not yet been identified.

All hormone receptors are specific cell structures that necessarily bind to hormones to show an effect. Receptors have high affinity and selectivity for hormones, but at the same time they can bind structural analogs of hormones. Therefore, in the literature it is common to speak of substances that mimic the action of a hormone - these are agonists, or mimetics, and substances that bind to receptors but do not cause a biological effect or prevent the binding of the hormone - antagonists, or lytics. Receptors are protein structures. They are synthesized in the endoplasmic reticulum in ribosomes. After formation, they undergo "maturation" in the Golgi apparatus, from where they are translocated to plasma membranes or to the cytosol.

The concentration of receptors on the cell surface depends on the level of hormones: if the concentration of a hormone in the blood increases, the number of receptors for this hormone on the membrane surface decreases - the sensitivity of the cell to this hormone decreases; if the level of a hormone in the blood decreases, the concentration of receptors for this hormone increases - the sensitivity of the cell to this hormone increases. This principle of regulation of the number of receptors is called down-regulation. For the interaction of a receptor with a hormone, the affinity of the hormone for that receptor is important, which depends on: 1) pH value - at acidification up to 7.0 the binding of insulin to insulin receptors decreases by 50%; 2) due to the appearance of autoantibodies (in conditions of pathology) to specific receptors. For example, in some forms of diabetes, despite the high level of insulin in the blood, there is a functional insufficiency of the insular apparatus - part of the insulin receptors is occupied by antibodies.

Mechanism of action of hormones. There are two main mechanisms of hormone action: 1) extracellular (action of protein hormones, catecholamines, serotonin, histamine) - in this case the receptors interacting with hormones are located on the membrane surface; 2) intracellular (action of steroid and thyroid hormones) - in this case hormones penetrate into the cytoplasm and interact with receptors located inside the cell. They are regulated by altering their synthesis. For example, during pregnancy in women, the concentration of oxytacin, serotonin, choline and adrenoreceptors in the myometrium changes significantly. These changes apparently occur under the influence of estrogens and progesterone.

Extracellular mechanism of hormone action. This mechanism can be visualized in the form of the following consecutive processes (p.56, Fig.Zh1): 1) interaction of the hormone and specific receptors with the formation of a hormone-receptor complex; 2) activation of the enzyme adenylate cyclase. This enzyme has regulatory and catalytic subunits. The regulatory subunit is associated with the hormone receptor. When a hormone is acted upon, the regulatory subunit is activated, which leads to an increase in the activity of the catalytic subunit, which is located on the inner side of the membrane; 3) synthesis of cAMP (3,5 cyclic adenosine monophosphate), which is accomplished by activation of the catalytic subunit of adenylate cyclase; 4) activation of protein kinase, or ATP-phosphotransferase (more specifically, cAMP-dependent protein kinase); and 5) the process of phosphorylation, which leads to the final physiological effect. For example, under the influence of ACTH, adrenal cells produce glucocorticoids. There are many varieties of protein kinases, with a different protein kinase for each protein. Signal transduction from the hormone-receptor complex to protein kinases is transmitted with the participation of specific mediators (secondary messengers). It has now been elucidated that such messengers can be: (a) cAMP (in the action of hormones ACTH, TTG, FSH, LH, ADH, catecholamines with beta effect, glucagon, paratgormone, calcitonin, secretin, thyreoliberin); b) calcium ions (in the action of hormones oxytocin, gastrin, cholicystokinin, angiotensin, catecholamines with alpha effect); c) diacylglycerol; d) secondary mediators of unknown nature (in the action of hormones STH, prolactin, somatostatin, insulin).

Messenger - calcium ions. Under the influence of hormones oxytocin, ADH, and gastrin, the content of calcium ions in the cell changes, and calcium ion-dependent protein kinases are activated. The activation process is associated with the interaction of calcium ions with the regulatory protein of the cell - calmodulin. Under resting conditions, this protein is in an inactive state. In the presence of calcium ions, calmedulin is activated, which leads to protein kinase activation, and further protein phosphorylation occurs. Thus, in this case, the sequence of cell activation processes can be visualized as follows: 1) formation of hormone-receptor complex; 2) increase of calcium level in the cell; 3) activation of calmodulin; 4) activation of protein kinase; 5) phosphorylation of regulator protein - increase of cell activity.

The messenger is diacylglycerol. Cell membranes contain phospholipids, in particular phosphatidylinositol - 4,5-biphosphate. When a hormone interacts with a receptor, this phospholipid ruptures to form diacylglycerol, which further activates protein kinase, resulting in phosphorylation of cell proteins.

Intracellular mechanism (action of steroid and thyroid hormones). In this case, the mechanism can be visualized in the form of the following sequential processes:

1) penetration of the hormone into the cytoplasm due to its lipophilicity and small size;

2) coupling of the hormone with specific receptor proteins (glucoprotein complexes);

3) disintegration of the glucoprotein complex;

4) penetration of the hormone-receptor complex into the nucleus;

5) the effect of the hormone on nuclear chromatin;

6) activation of the transcription process (induction of matrix RNA);

7) activation (simultaneously) of RNA polymerase and synthesis of ribosomal RNA - an additional number of ribosomes is formed, which bind to the membranes of the endoplasmic reticulum. Thus, in the

intracellular mechanism, 2-3 hours after exposure to the hormone, enhanced protein synthesis is observed.

Regulation of hormone secretion: 1) hormonal regulation through the production of liberins and statins in the hypothalamus, which through the portal system of the pituitary gland from the hypothalamus reach the adenohypophysis (anterior lobe) and enhance (liberins) or inhibit (statins) the production of the corresponding hormones. The hypothalamus produces 7 liberins and 3 statins (corticoliberin, thyreoliberin, foliberin, luliberin, melanoliberin, prolactoliberin, somatoliberin, somatostatin, melanostatin, and prolactostatin). Adenohypophysis hormones in turn cause changes in the production of hormones of the corresponding glands of internal secretion; 2) regulation of hormone production by the feedback principle. For example, the production of thyroid hormones of the thyroid gland is regulated by thyreoliberin of the hypothalamus, affecting the adenohypophysis, producing thyroid hormone (TTH), which increases the production of thyroid hormones. Once in the blood, thyroid hormones act on the hypothalamus and adenohypophysis and inhibit (if the level of thyroid hormones is high) the production of thyreoliberin and TTH; 3) regulation with the participation of CNS structures: sympathetic and parasympathetic nervous systems cause changes in hormone production. Activation of the sympathetic section of the ANS leads to increased production of adrenaline in the brain layer of the adrenal glands, and increase of the parasympathetic section leads to increased production of insulin. Different structures of the hypothalamus cause changes in hormone production. Emotional, mental influences through the structures of the limbic system, through hypothalamic formations can significantly affect the activity of cells producing hormones.

Destruction of hormones (catabolism). Hormones are broken down very rapidly in tissues, particularly in the liver. The half-life of a hormone (the time it takes to break down half of the available hormone) ranges from a few minutes to two hours.

There are several types of interaction between endocrine glands: 1) interaction according to the principle of positive and negative direct and feedback. For example, TTG stimulates the production of thyroid hormones. When the anterior lobe of the pituitary gland is removed, thyroid atrophy occurs - this direct positive relationship. Hyperfunction of the thyroid gland inhibits the formation of TTG - negative feedback; 2) synergism of hormonal influences, or unidirectional action of different hormones. For example, adrenaline (adrenal medulla) and glucagon (pancreas) - activate the breakdown of glycogen in the liver to glucose and cause an increase in blood sugar; 3) Antagonism of hormonal influences. For example, insulin and adrenaline cause different effects: insulin - hypoglycemia (due to increased penetration of glucose to cells with the further process of its utilization), adrenaline - hyperglycemia (due to conversion of reserve liver glycogen into glucose, which enters the blood); 4) permissive (permissive) action of hormones, which is expressed in the fact that the hormone itself does not cause a physiological effect, but creates a condition for the reaction of cells and tissues to the action of other hormones. For example, the action of glucocorticoids on the effects of adrenaline. Glucocorticoids themselves do not affect vascular tone, but they create conditions under which even subthreshold concentrations of adrenaline increase BP and cause hyperglycemia as a result of glucogenolysis in the liver.

Lecture 27.

<u>Topic: Hormones of the posterior and intermediate lobes of the pituitary gland. The role of the epiphysis. The importance of the thymus, thyroid and perithyroid glands.</u>

Objective - To know the role of hormones of the posterior and intermediate lobe of the pituitary, epiphysis, thymus, thyroid and parathyroid glands.

The objectives are.

(a) Discover the role of hormones of the posterior and intermediate lobe of the pituitary and epiphysis;

b) show the role of the thymus in immunologic functions;

c) indicate the role of thyroid hormones on oxidative processes and heat production;

d) give the role of perithyroid hormones in the regulation of calcium and phosphorus metabolism.

Content:

Kvetnoy I.M., Konovalov S.S. in the book "Magic Molecules of Health" compare the endocrine system of the body to an orchestra performing a symphony of life: "Endocrine cells located in different organs and producing different hormones make up an orchestra performing a symphony of life. The cells and the hormones they produce are the instruments of the endocrine orchestra. They are led by a very experienced and strict conductor - the hypothalamus. His right hand and faithful assistant, the conductor of all his ideas and aspirations - the pituitary gland. The pituitary gland is connected with the hypothalamus by a system of special communication: nerve fibers and blood vessels".

Epiphysis, or pineal gland. The epiphysis looks like a small spruce cone, so it was named the pineal gland, which in humans weighs 0.1 grams and is three to four millimeters in diameter. Four thousand years ago, Indian yogis gave a name to this gland - "pineal gland". They believed that the function of this gland was for clairvoyance and reflection on previous incarnations of the spirit. René Descartes in the 17th century called this gland the "receptacle of the soul". The function of the epiphysis was unclear for a long time. In the late 50s of the twentieth century, American dermatologist A. Lerner drew attention to an article by British scientists C. McCord and F. Allen, published in 1917, which reported on the brightening of the color of the body of tadpoles when feeding them extracts of epiphysis. A. Lerner searched for effective cosmetic brightening agents for the treatment of pigmented dermatoses. He attracted the famous American biochemist Julius Axelrod to his work. Through the efforts of biochemists, dermatologists and endocrinologists, tens of thousands of bovine pineal glands were processed and several grams of a substance with a powerful brightening effect on frog skin were obtained. This is how the epiphysis hormone **melatonin was** discovered. D. Axelrod was awarded the Nobel Prize in 1970. Further research showed that the immediate precursor of melatonin is **serotonin**. It was found that the concentration of melatonin increases at night, which leads to a decrease in the concentration of serotonin, and vice versa during the day. Serotonin deficiency in brain tissue, even when its level in serum is high enough, is a pathogenetic factor in the development of depression. Melatonin and serotonin have a wide spectrum of action: they control pigment metabolism, sexual functions (inhibits the production of gonadoliberins in the hypothalamus, the consequence of which is the inhibition of gonadotropic hormone production in the anterior lobe of the pituitary gland), circadian and seasonal rhythms, the processes of cell division and differentiation, participate in the formation of visual perception of images and color perception, sleep and wakefulness. It has been established that the concentration of melatonin in the blood serum of cancer patients sharply increases 1.5-2 times compared to the norm, and in case of metastasis it sharply decreases. The product of melatonin reduction is **adrenoglomerulotropin** - this hormone was discovered by Farell (1960) - this hormone stimulated aldosterone secretion in decerebrated dogs, but had no effect on intact animals. Farell explained this by the fact that the epiphysis produces two hormones that affect the electrolyte composition of the blood: **adrenoglomerulotropin,** which stimulates the production of aldosterone and increases the reabsorption of sodium ions in the tubules of the nephron and **anticorticotropin,** which inhibits the secretion of aldosterone. Biochemists have found that the epiphysis produces another hormone, **antihypothalamic factor, which prevents the** hypothalamus from reaching the threshold of its activity and thus prevents the onset of old age.

The hypothalamus is the central control organ of the endocrine system. Scientists have found that the activity of the hypothalamus increases throughout life. According to modern ideas, aging processes, serious age-related cardiovascular disorders, and tumor growth are the result of the hypothalamus reaching a certain threshold of its activity. The supraoptic and paraventricular nuclei of the hypothalamus produce antidiuretic hormone (ADH) and oxytocin, which are accumulated in the accumulating Herrings' corpuscles of the neurohypophysis (posterior lobe of the pituitary gland). From here, these hormones enter the bloodstream. ADH acts on the collecting tubes of the nephron and activates the enzyme hyaluronidase, which breaks down hyaluronic acid, which leads to an increase in the pores in the collecting tubes due to which water reabsorption increases, oliguria occurs, and at high concentrations of ADH anuria may occur. On the other hand, due to water reabsorption, osmotic pressure of blood decreases, ICP increases due to the liquid part, which leads to a decrease in hematocrit. Since at high concentrations ADH increases the contraction of vascular SMCs, which leads to an increase in pressure, therefore ADH is also called vasopressin. Oxytocin plays the role of a regulator of uterine activity and participates in the processes of lactation, increasing milk secretion by activating myoepithelial cells. Increased production of oxytocin occurs under the influence of impulses from the receptors of the cervix, as well as under the influence of irritation of mechanoreceptors of the nipples of the mammary gland, which occurs during breastfeeding.

The pituitary gland is a lower brain appendage located at the base of the skull at the bottom of the Turkish saddle. In humans, this organ weighs 0.6 g. According to modern nomenclature, the pituitary gland has two main parts: adenohypophysis and neurohypophysis. The adenohypophysis, or glandular part is divided into three lobes: anterior, tuberal and intermediate. The posterior lobe of the neurohypophysis is closely connected with the hypothalamus. Fibers of the hypothalamic-pituitary tract, coming from the supraoptic and paraventricular nuclei, end there.

The anterior lobe of the pituitary gland has a close vascular connection with the hypothalamus. The anterior lobe is the largest part of the adenohypophysis. The anterior lobe of the pituitary gland produces 7 tropic hormones, as these hormones regulate the function of the peripheral endocrine glands. These include: adrenocorticotropic hormone (ACTH), thyroid hormone (TTH), luteinizing hormone (LH), follicle stimulating hormone (FSH), somatotropic hormone (STH), lipotropins, and prolactin. **ACTH** affects the adrenal cortex and increases corticosteroid release. The influence of the pituitary gland on the adrenal cortex was first established by Ascoli and Lignein in 1912 in experiments on pituitary-ectomized dogs. **TTH** affects the thyroid gland and enhances thyroxine release. The biological properties of TTH are that it causes changes in the morphology and function of the thyroid gland - increasing its size and blood flow, increasing iodine accumulation, activating the biosynthesis of thyroid hormones and releasing them into the bloodstream. The ability of the pituitary gland to influence the function of the sex glands was established by Aschner in 1912. In experiments on pituitaryectomized dogs, atrophy of the sex glands and secondary sexual characteristics was observed. It was found that there are two gonadotropic origins in the pituitary gland, **follicle-stimulating hormone (FSH) and luteinizing hormone (LH).** **LH** acts on the corpus luteum and increases the production of progesterone. Increased concentration of LH in the blood promotes the process of ovulation. Under its influence, the follicle wall ruptures, and in place of the burst follicle is formed functionally active corpus luteum. LH is also inherent stimulating effect on the interstitial tissue of the ovaries and testes. LH stimulates the formation of estrogens in women and androgens in men. **FSH** in women acts on the ovaries, accelerating oocyte growth and development, and in men acts on the testes, accelerating sperm growth and development. For these effects of FSH to occur, small amounts of LH or estrogen in the ovaries and testosterone in the testes must be present. **Prolactin, or luteotropic hormone (LTP)** stimulates mammary gland growth and promotes milk formation. This hormone stimulates the synthesis of the protein, lacalbumin, fats and carbohydrates in milk. Prolactin also stimulates the formation of the corpus luteum and its production of progesterone. This hormone stimulates milk formation, increasing the synthesis of milk proteins, has an antigonadotropic effect - inhibits the production and release of FSH and LH. STH affects the liver and somatomedins are formed, which act on organs and tissues, increasing protein synthesis, promoting growth and development of tissues. Human height increases before the age of 25 and remains constant until the age of 60 and decreases by 2-3 cm by the age of 70. According to WHO, the average height for women is 160 cm and for men 170 cm. Figures below 145 cm and above 195 cm is considered pathology and is associated with a violation of the synthesis of growth hormone - STH. The first assumption about the presence of growth hormone in the pituitary gland was made in 1921 by American scientists H. Evans and G. Long. In 1964-1968, scientist S. Lee managed to isolate STH in the form of a purified preparation by processing 200 thousand bovine pituitary glands. Hypofunction of the pituitary gland leads to dwarfism, a hereditary disease. They are found to have short stature at birth (20 to 38 cm, with a weight of 500-1500 grams. This pathology is called pituitary nanism (from the Greek word nanos - dwarf), in life these people are called midgets. They have preserved all the proportions of the body and in the future their development proceeds quite normally. The increase in human growth can be twofold and depends on the age at which pituitary hyperfunction occurs. If pituitary hyperfunction is noted in a child's body, gigantism occurs - there is a proportional increase in all parts of the body. People-giants reach a height of 2.5 meters. Their life expectancy is inversely proportional to body size. People over 230 cm rarely live longer than 35 years. If hyperfunction of the pituitary gland occurs in adulthood, acromegaly (from Greek akron - limb, megas - large) occurs. In adulthood, the epiphyseal (sprouting) cartilages of the bones are already closed and therefore the length of the skeleton does not change. Body weight gain is only at the expense of soft tissues: muscles, fatty fiber, skin. This pathology was first described by French physician P. Marie in 1896, describing in his words "terrible" patient: general obesity, the head is enlarged in size, facial features are coarse, nose is enlarged, lips are thickened, the face is swollen, eyes "come out" of the orbits, the tongue does not fit in the mouth, limbs (especially hands) are enlarged, fingers have a characteristic sausage shape.

Lipotropins promote mobilization of fat from fat depots and induce lipolysis with an increase in unesterified fatty acids in the blood.

Intermediate lobe of the pituitary gland - melanocytostimulating hormone is produced here, which regulates changes in skin coloration. This hormone was first named intermedin by Tsondek, then Lerner proposed the term melanocytostimulating hormone (MSH) because this hormone affects melanocytes in the skin. An increase in MSH concentration causes an increase in free melatonin in the epidermis surrounding the melanocytes. Thus MSH stimulates the dispersion and synthesis of melatonin in human skin. When there is a high concentration of MSH in the blood, the skin becomes bronzed (Adison's disease). MSH production is regulated through the hypothalamus by melanostatin, which inhibits MSH production.

Posterior lobe of the pituitary gland, or neurohypophysis - two hormones are produced here: vasopressin or antidiuretic hormone (ADH) and oxytocin. Pure oxytocin was first obtained from the neurohypophysis in 1949 (Livermore, du Vigneaud). Vasopressin increases the activity of vascular SMCs, causing vasoconstriction. Vasopressin also acts on the collecting tube of the nephron, increasing the activity of the enzyme hyaluronidase in it. This enzyme breaks down hyaluronic acid in the wall of the collecting tube and enlarges the pores resulting in increased water reabsorption and decreased diuresis, hence the second name for vasopressin, ADH. The increase in water reabsorption through the rotary countercurrent mechanism increases the reabsorption of sodium ions. Thus vasopressin is involved in water and salt metabolism. Oxytocin increases the contraction of the uterus (involved in the regulation of labor) and the musculature of the alveoli of the mammary gland, increasing milk secretion.

The goiter gland, or thymus gland **(the upper arches of this gland have the form of a fork)** - weight on average 10-15 g (0.5% of the weight), the maximum is reached by 11-15 years (30-40 g), and with the onset of puberty thymus gland begins to slowly atrophy, by 40 years of age reaches a weight of 3 g (0.005% of the weight), that is, with age the weight of the thymus decreases by 100 times. The thymus gland hormone thymosin was isolated in 1968 by Goldstein et al. This hormone stimulates lymphocyte proliferation. After removal of the thymus gland in animals, a decrease in the number of lymphocytes in the blood, lymph nodes and spleen is found. The role of the thymus gland in erythropoiesis is known. Thymomas are known to be accompanied by aplastic anemia (absence of reticulocytes in the peripheral blood and erythroblasts in the bone marrow). In 1961, Miller's article "The Immunologic Function of the Thymus" appears, in which he showed that the thymus is the main organ of immunity. Lymphocytes arise in the thymus during the newborn period. Miller found that the removal of the thymus in newborn mice causes pathology described as wasting-syndrome (from English wasting - exhaustion): growth retardation, baldness, intestinal disorders, "thinning" of the blood due to a decrease in red blood cells, leukocytes and platelets, there are severe immunological disorders. At the same time, any infection can be fatal. According to Burnet (1964), the differentiation of lymphocytes (T-lymphocytes) for specific immunologic functions occurs in the thymus. Of the many biologically active substances (21), three hormones have been most studied: thymosin, thymine, and T-activin. Thymosin stimulates lymphocyte development. Thymine acts on muscle tissue. In this case, antibodies are produced that interact with the H-cholinoreactive structure of muscle and acetylcholine does not act on the postsynaptic membrane, which inhibits neuromuscular transmission, causing muscle atrophy - myasthenia gravis occurs, which is manifested by muscle weakness and rapid muscle fatigue, observed in hyperfunction of the thymus gland. These symptoms go away after thymectomy. T-activin has the same properties as thymine, but is 6-9 times more active. In St. Petersburg Institute of Bioregulation and Gerontology under the direction of V.Kh Khavinson was created thymus preparation thymogen, on the basis of which was synthesized vilon, which has geroprotective properties: slows down aging of cells, tissues, organs and prolongs the life of experimental animals. Studies of various aspects of thymus activity have become so broad that the term "thymology" - the science of thymus - appeared in the literature.

Thyroid gland - produces thyroid hormones in the blood: iodine-containing amino acids thyroxine and triiodotyrosine, which influence the basic functions of the body - growth, development and metabolism. The main thyroid hormone is thyroxine, which makes up ¾ of all blood iodine. In the circulation in small quantities is triiodotyrosine. Under the influence of thyroid hormones, growth, absorption of oxygen, various aspects of metabolism and the activity of individual enzyme systems are altered. It has been found that with the removal of the thyroid gland in animals and hypothyroidism in humans comes a delay in growth and development of the body. Thyroid hormones increase the processes of oxygen uptake and heat formation. This is due to the fact that in hyperfunction of the thyroid gland sharply increases the basic metabolism, exceeding the level of proper basic metabolism over the actual. The role of the thyroid gland in the regulation of water metabolism in the body is known. Thus, polyuria in patients with hyperthyroidism and oliguria in patients with hypothyroidism are noted. Thyroid hormones affect nitrogen metabolism (under the action of thyroxine in healthy people there is a negative nitrogen balance), which is confirmed by an increase in nitrogen excretion with urine. Thyroid hormones have a significant effect on all phases of carbohydrate transformation in the body, accelerate the absorption of glucose in the GI tract, participate in the regulation of blood sugar levels, intervening in the processes of glucose breakdown, glycogen synthesis in the liver. Thyroid hormones act on lipid metabolism: thyroid hypofunction is always accompanied by an increase in blood cholesterol, neutral fats and phospholipids. The mechanism of action of thyroid hormones is associated with its direct action on the metabolism of substances and energy in mitochondria. In addition, thyroid hormones stimulate protein and DNA biosynthesis. Thus, these hormones on two targets in the cell: one at the level of the nucleus and the other at the level of the mitochondria. When iodine intake is reduced, hypothyroidism sets in. In basal disease (due to thyroid hyperfunction), there is weight loss, profuse sweating, diarrhea, and lack of skin infiltration. If hypofunction of the thyroid gland in childhood, there is a delay in growth, violation of body proportions, sexual and mental development - such a pathological condition is called cretinism. In adults, hypofunction of the thyroid gland leads to a pathological condition - myxedema, or Shimomoto's disease. In such patients, an increase in body weight occurs due to an increase in the amount of tissue fluid and puffiness of the face. These processes are associated with the accumulation of albumin in the tissue fluid resulting in an increase in the oncotic pressure of the tissue fluid. Hyperthyroidism is rarely due to excess iodine, as it is well excreted by the kidneys. The cause of hyperthyroidism becomes a pathology of the pituitary gland, which is accompanied by an increase in the production of TTH, which accelerates the synthesis of thyroxine in the thyroid gland. Most often the cause is hereditary predisposition or tumor.

The perithyroid glands, or parathyroid glands, were first described as separate entities by Sandstrom in 1880. McCallum and Fetlin in 1908 noted that tetany following removal of the parathyroid glands is associated with impaired calcium metabolism. Four parathyroid glands, weighing 0.3 grams in total, are usually noted. They produce two hormones: parathormone and calcitonin. Being antagonists, they regulate phosphorus-calcium metabolism. Paratgormone increases blood calcium levels and decreases phosphorus concentrations. Calcitonin has the opposite effect: it decreases calcium and increases phosphorus accumulation. Tumors can occur in the parathyroid gland - parathyroid adenoma. The tumor consists of cells that produce calcitonin. This disease was first described by the German pathologist F. Recklinghausen in 1891. Recklinghausen's disease is a systemic bone disease based on disorders of calcium and phosphorus metabolism due to hyperfunction of parathyroid glands associated with adenoma or hyperplasia of these glands and is characterized by impoverishment of bone tissue with calcium salts (skeletal decalcinosis) due to calcium leaching from bones and increased excretion of calcium by urine. The bones become first flexible, then brittle. In this regard, spontaneous multiple fractures of bones (limbs, ribs and vertebrae) may occur. In the early stages of the disease sharply increases the mobility of the joints, patients can take unnatural postures (put your legs behind your head, twisting spiral. As the disease progresses, there is a disfiguring deformation of the skeleton, loss of teeth, kidney stones are formed.

Lecture 28.

Topic: Endocrine function of the pancreas, adrenal and sex glands. Endocrine function of the placenta. The female menstrual cycle.

Objective - to know the main influences of pancreatic, adrenal, sex glands and placental hormones.

The objectives are.

(a) Show the role of pancreatic hormones in the regulation of metabolism;

b) reveal the role of adrenal cortex hormones (mineralocorticoids, glucocorticoids, sex hormones) and brain matter (adrenaline and noradrenaline) in the processes of adaptation of the organism;

c) indicate the role of male and female sex hormones in the formation of sex and the regulation of reproduction;

d) give the characteristics of the function of the sex glands during the female menstrual cycle.

Content:

The endocrine part of the pancreas is represented by groups of light-colored cells located among exocrine tissue and called **islets of Langerhans.** Currently, three types of cells are distinguished: alpha, beta and delta. In most mammals, the number of beta cells is 3-4 times higher than alpha cells. Delta cells make up about 5% of the total mass of the islets of Langerhans and produce somatostatin and regulate the activity of alpha cells. **Insulin.** Bunting and Best in 1922 isolated an extract from the pancreas that eliminated hyperglycemia and glucosuria. In 1925 Abel obtained crystalline insulin, which is a protein of small molecular weight, from this extract. Insulin is formed by beta cells. Shortly after the introduction of insulin into clinical practice, it was noted that after its intravenous injections, its characteristic hypoglycemic action is preceded by a brief hyperglycemia. Subsequently it became known that the hyperglycemia was induced by another substance contained in the pancreatic extract. Murlin et al. (1923) named this substance **glucagon, or sugar mobilizer.** Staub et al. in 1953 obtained a pure crystalline preparation of glucagon. Glucagon is formed in the alpha cells of the islets of Langerhans. The main physiological effect of glucagon is to increase blood glucose levels by increasing glycogenolysis in the liver. The hyperglycemic effect may be due to stimulation of adrenaline secretion, which also increases glycogen breakdown in the liver. In addition, glucagon actively stimulates gluconeogenesis. It has a lipolytic effect.

Adrenal glands - the first description of the adrenal glands was made in 1563 by Bartholomew Eustachius. There is an assumption that Leonardo da Vinci described the adrenal glands in 1510. Addison started talking about the function of the adrenal glands in 1856, when he made the first attempt to link the clinical symptoms of the disease, which was accompanied by sharp weakness, gauntness, bronze coloring of the skin, with a violation of the adrenal glands. The weight of the adrenal glands in humans is 4 to 14 grams. - Men are 30% larger than women. Between 1933 and 1953, corticosterone, dehydrocorticosterone, dehydrocorticosterone, hydrocortisone, deoxycorticosterone, and the most potent mineralocorticoid aldosterone were isolated from adrenal extracts in crystalline form. Between 1937 and 1944, deoxycorticosterone, corticosterone were synthesized, and in 1950. - The synthesis of hydrocortisone. The most active mineralocorticoid is aldosterone, which causes retention of sodium and chlorine ions in the body and increased excretion of potassium, hydrogen, ammonium, calcium, and magnesium. **Adrenal** medullary **substance** (medullary substance, adrenal tissue) - is located in the center of the gland and makes up its smaller part. For the first time the role of hormones of the adrenal medullary layer is evidenced by the works of Oliver and Schiffer, conducted in 1894. They found that extracts of this tissue introduced into the blood increase blood pressure. In 1901 Aldrich and independently Takamine isolated from adrenal tissue the active substance, which they called epinephrine or adrenaline. Later Euler discovered noradrenaline in the medullary layer of the adrenal gland, which differs from adrenaline by the absence of a methyl grouping. Then dopamine was discovered. All the hormones of the brain layer of the adrenal gland are derivatives of pyrocatechin - they are called catecholamines. Adrenaline and noradrenaline have been found to have numerous effects like the sympathetic nervous system: activation of cardiac activity, increase in vascular tone, relaxation of bronchial smooth muscle, etc. Catecholamines have an effect on the CCC. Adrenaline effectively affects carbohydrate metabolism: causes hyperglycemia, reduces the content of glycogen in the liver and skeletal muscles, promotes the accumulation of lactic acid, activates phosphorylase. The mechanism of hyperglycemia is that adrenaline accelerates glycogen breakdown on the one hand and depresses synthesis on the other. In addition, catecholamines reduce glucose uptake by tissues and depress hexokinase activity. Adrenaline and noradrenaline have a pronounced effect on fat metabolism. There is a significant mobilization of fatty acids and an increase in their content in the blood. Under the influence of catecholamines, lipase of adipose tissue is activated and oxidation of fatty acids increases. Catecholamines participate in the activation of thermogenesis.

Adrenal cortex - the adrenal cortex has three zones: the outer - tubular, middle - fascicular and inner - reticular. Mineralocorticoids are produced in the tubular zone, glucocorticoids are produced in the bundle zone, and sex hormones, mainly androgens, are produced in the reticular zone. The main representative of **mineralocorticoids is aldosterone,** which acts on the ascending rectal tubule and increases the reabsorption of sodium ions, then through the pivotally countercurrent system increases the reabsorption of water. The mechanism of active reabsorption of sodium ions is coupled with the opposite process of removal of potassium ions from the blood into the terminal urine. Enhancement of aldosterone production is due to angiotensin-II. The second mechanism of regulation of aldosterone production is the hormone of the anterior lobe of the pituitary gland ACTH, but in this case the release of aldosterone is much less. The third mechanism is through the direct effect of sodium and potassium on aldosterone-producing cells. Among the various **glucocorticoids, the** most important are **cortisol, cortisone, and corticosterone.** Cortisol has the strongest physiologic effect. Glucocorticoids cause: 1) increase in blood glucose content due to activation of gluconeogenesis: formation of glucose from amino acids and fatty acids; 2) activation of lipolysis. Thus, glucocorticoids contribute to the mobilization of energy resources of the body. In addition, glucocorticoids depress all components of the inflammatory response and sharply reduce the number of lymphocytes. Glucocorticoids increase the sensitivity of vascular smooth muscle to catecholamines. In low concentrations glucocorticoids cause an increase in diuresis - by increasing the rate of glomerular filtration and inhibition of ADH release. At high concentrations, glucocorticoids behave like aldosterone. Glucocorticoids increase hydrochloric acid and pepsin secretion.

Glucocorticoid release is regulated by **corticoliberin and ACTH.** Corticoliberin is formed in the hypothalamus and acts on the anterior lobe of the pituitary gland, increasing the release of ACTH, which acts on the bundle zone of the adrenal cortex and increases the release of glucocorticoids. Hypofunction of the adrenal cortex is manifested by a decrease in the content of corticoid hormones and is called Addison's (bronze) disease. In this case, there is adynamia, decreased CCA, arterial hypotension, hypoglycemia, increased skin pigmentation, diarrhea. In adrenal tumors can occur hyperfunction of the adrenal cortex with an increase in glucocorticoids - hypercorticism, or Icenko-Cushing's syndrome. **Sex hormones** play a role only during childhood. These hormones contribute to the development of secondary sexual characteristics. ACTH stimulates the synthesis and secretion of androgens. In the absence of an enzyme involved in the formation of cortisol, ACTH synthesis increases, leading to an increase in androgen concentration - adrenogenital syndrome: female development in the male type.

Reninangiotensin system. This system includes renin, angiotensinogen, angiotensin-I, angiotensin-II, and angiotensin-III. This system contributes to the self-regulation of homeostasis of the internal environment by normalizing the amount of fluid, sodium ions, and blood pressure. Angiotensinogen is a protein (alpha-2 globulin) that is synthesized in the liver. The enzyme renin is synthesized in the kidneys and facilitates the conversion of angiotensinogen to angiotensin-I by cleaving the amino acid chain resulting in a decapeptide (of 10 amino acids). Under the influence of another enzyme - carboxydipeptidyl peptidase (converting enzyme) from angiotensin-I (decapeptide), two more amino acids are cleaved and an octapeptide (of 8 amino acids) is formed - angiotensin-II - one of the powerful vasoconstrictors. This substance has the following mechanisms of action: 1) activates vascular SMCs, causing vasoconstriction (vasoconstriction) and an increase in blood pressure; 2) activates aldosterone production, contributing to increased reabsorption of sodium ions, which through a turn-over-countercurrent mechanism increases water reabsorption; 3) increases production of vasopressin (antidiuretic hormone - ADH), which on the one hand causes activation of vascular SMCs and vasoconstriction and on the other hand ADH increases water reabsorption in collecting tubes. Thus, angiotensin-II contributes to BP increase by increasing resistance (due to vasoconstriction) and volume velocity (volume of fluid flowing in vessels) by increasing water reabsorption. Renin is produced in juxtaglomerular cells surrounding the bringing arteriole of the renal tubule. Renin production is accomplished by the following mechanisms: 1) when blood pressure in the bringing arteriole decreases; 2) via the sympathetic nerve of the ANS, with norepinephrine interacting with the beta-1 adrenergic subunit of these cells; and 3) when blood sodium ion levels decrease, renin production increases. It is believed that from angiotensin-II by cleavage of arginine a septapeptide (of 7 amino acids) - angiotensin-III is formed, which has increased affinity to the receptors of the adrenal cortex.

Kallikrein-kinin system. In addition to angiotensinogen activation, alpha-2 globulins are a humoral factor in the regulation of kinins (peptides), among which bradykinin (9 amino acids) and lysylbradykinin or kallidin (10 amino acids) are of particular importance. Tissue and plasma kllikrein, which are in an inactive state, prekallikrein, participate in the formation of bradykinin. Plasmin is involved in the activation of prekallikrein. Bradykinin is formed in the following way: under the influence of tissue kallikrein enzyme (kininogenase) from plasma alpha-2 globulin kallidin is detached from which, under the influence of plasma kallikrein amino acid arginine is detached and bradykinin is formed. Bradykinin is an antagonist of anihyotensin because it relaxes the SMCs, i.e. it is a vasodilator - one of the strongest vasodilators. In addition, bradykinin increases capillary permeability and causes fluid to leave the vessel (edema occurs). Under normal conditions, bradykinin in large quantities is formed in sweat and salivary glands, which contributes to the expansion of blood vessels and increased fluid output, which is important for sweat and salivation. Under the influence of kininase bradykinin undergoes inactivation.

Gonads - testes (testis) and ovaries (ovarium) are organs that produce spermatozoa and eggs. In inseparable connection with this gametogenic function of the gonads is their hormonal activity, so the testes and ovaries are considered to be endocrine glands. The main role of sex hormones is to ensure the normal course of the function of reproduction. Sex hormones affect the maturation of gametes, cause structural and biochemical changes in the organs of the sexual sphere, aimed at preserving the viability, activation and transport of gametes in the genital tract, create conditions for fertilization of the egg and its implantation in the uterus. The hormones of the sex glands during periods corresponding to the appearance of the mature ovum affect the hypothalamus and cause changes in sexual behavior. The role of the sex glands on the genitals was first established by A. Berthold in 1849 when transplanting rooster testes to a capoon. Further studies established that the removal of sex glands in male and female animals caused atrophy of the penis, prostate, cessation of sperm production, involution of the crest in roosters. In female and female animals ovariectomy caused atrophy of uterus, vagina, mammary glands, and implantation of gonads restored the structure of these organs. The first preparations of pure hormones were isolated from urine. In 1934-1938, estradiol and testosterone were isolated from extracts of the sex glands and were much more active than their urinary metabolites. Sexual gland hormones are divided into steroidal and peptide hormones according to their chemical structure.

Peptide hormones. Relaxin - is formed by cells of the corpus luteum, causes relaxation of the ligaments of the bosom articulation, reduces the tone of the uterus and its contractility. This effect is enhanced against the background of increased concentration of estrogen. **Inhibin -** produced by the cells of the seminal tubules of the testes. In the presence of this hormone reduces the production of FSH in the anterior lobe of the pituitary gland. Inhibin is also found in the follicular fluid of the ovaries.

Steroid hormones. These hormones are produced by the sex glands. Male sex hormones (androgens) are produced in the testes and provide androgenization of the body. Female sex hormones (estrogens and progesterones) are produced in the ovaries and corpus luteum and provide feminization of the body. It should be noted that androgens are produced in small quantities in the ovaries and estrogens in the testes.

Estrogens - their synthesis is carried out in ovarian follicles, their specific action is aimed at the development of organs of the female genital sphere, they are necessary for the normal development of follicles, strengthen the effect of FSH on the ovaries. Estrogens maintain the viability of oocytes. In the mammary glands, estrogens cause proliferation, with ductal growth mainly occurring. The hormone FSH is required for estrogens to act on the mammary glands. **Progesterone** is the hormone of pregnancy preservation and is produced in the ovarian corpus luteum, which develops in place of a burst follicle. Progesterone promotes the development of the endometrial glands - the glands secrete large amounts of secretion containing glycogen, mucoproteins, salts, which serve as a nourishing environment for the zygote before the formation of the placenta. Under the influence of progesterone, there is further development of blood vessels of the endometrium. Progesterone has the opposite effect of estrogen on the myometrium: there is a relaxation of muscle fibers, which contributes to their stretching as pregnancy progresses, reduces the excitability of the myometrium and weakens the effect of oxytocin. Progesterone stimulates the development of mammary gland alveoli after the preliminary action of estrogen. Progesterone inhibits the onset of lactogenesis by inhibition of prolactin release from the pituitary gland. The effect of progesterone on the hypothalamus is accompanied by an increase in body temperature.

Placenta. The placenta provides nutrition to the embryo and is a temporary endocrine gland of the body during pregnancy. Placental hormones determine the tone of the smooth muscle of the uterus, serve to preserve pregnancy, provide the processes of mammogenesis. The protein hormones of the placenta include: chorionic gonadotropin (CG) and placental lactogenic hormone (PLH). The maximum secretion of CG is observed at 7-12 weeks of pregnancy and then decreases. This hormone stimulates progesterone synthesis in the corpus luteum during the early stages of pregnancy. CH has follicle-stimulating activity, causing the maturation of follicles and the synthesis of estrogen in them. PLG in many properties is an analog of pituitary STG and contributes to the enhancement of its action. Production of PLH is insignificant at the beginning of pregnancy and progressively increases towards the end of pregnancy. PLH increases protein synthesis in the maternal body. Steroid hormones (pregnenolone and progesterone) are synthesized from cholesterol by active enzymatic systems of the placenta. During pregnancy, the amount of progesterone increases dramatically. Progesterone production up to 4-6 weeks of pregnancy is carried out by the corpus luteum, but from 5-7 weeks the placenta is actively involved in this process. During pregnancy, the secretion of progesterone increases 10-fold.

The menstrual cycle ensures the integration of various processes necessary for reproductive function: oocyte maturation and ovulation, periodic preparation of the endometrium for implantation of a fertilized egg. A distinction is made between ovarian and uterine cycles. On average, the menstrual cycle lasts 28 days (variations from 21 days to 32 days are possible). The ovarian cycle consists of three phases: 1) follicular (day 1 through day 14 of the cycle). In this phase, the amount of estrogen predominates, the maximum concentration of which reaches 1 day before ovulation; 2) ovulatory phase (day 13 of the cycle). In this phase, the concentration of lutinizing hormone increases, the maximum concentration of which reaches during ovulation; 3) luteal phase (from day 15 to 28). In this phase, the concentration of progesterone predominates. The uterine cycle consists of 4 phases: 1) desquamation (duration of 3-5 days); 2) regeneration (up to day 5-6 of the cycle); 3) proliferation (up to day 14) - provided by estrogen, in this phase there is a thickening of the endometrial mucosa and the development of its glands; 4) secretion (from day 15 to 28) - provided by the increasing concentration of progesterone. In the first days of the menstrual cycle under the influence of FSH follicle maturation occurs, which leads to an increase in the concentration of estrogen. The increase in estrogen concentration is also affected by luteinizing hormone. In the middle of the cycle sharply increases the concentration of LH, which leads to ovulation. After ovulation, the concentration of progesterone rises sharply and by feedback inhibits the secretion of FSH and LH, which prevents the maturation of a new follicle. Degeneration of the corpus luteum occurs. Estrogen and progesterone levels fall.

Androgens. The most active of them is testosterone. Other androgens - androstenedione, androsterone have 6-10 times less activity, and such androgens as dihydroepiandrosmterone, epitestosterone - 25-50 times less activity. The role of testosterones during the fetal period (from the 12th to the 23rd week) is in the sexual differentiation of the organism. During this period, the fetal testes secrete testosterone intensively, ensuring sexual differentiation of the hypothalamus, as well as the formation of internal and external genitalia in the male type, which contributes to the genotypic sex to form into phenotypic sex. The physiologic role of androgens in the male body is to stimulate certain stages of spermatogenesis and the development of secondary sexual characteristics. Androgens enlarge the larynx and increase the thickness of the vocal cords, resulting in a lowered voice. Androgens have a powerful anabolic effect, which is associated with the stimulation of protein synthesis, due to which the muscle develops. During puberty, the anabolic effect of androgens leads to increased growth (pubertal growth spurt), and then androgens cause the epiphyseal cartilages to close and eventually growth ceases. In the female body, the role of androgens is the need for protein synthesis in the organs of the reproductive system. With prolonged action of an increased amount of androgens in the female body degeneration of mammary glands and female secondary sexual characteristics with the development of masculinization (hair growth of the male type, coarsening of the voice, development of musculature). When acting on the preoptic centers of the hypothalamus androgens cause the appearance of male sexual behavior and the development of aggression, in women this role is performed by estrogens. The maximum production of androgens by the sex glands in men is observed at the age of 25-35 years. In most men high levels of testosterone is maintained until 60-70 years, then steeply declines and at the age of 80 years there is a very low level of testosterone in the blood. The regulation of testosterone synthesis is through LH. Testosterone stimulates erythropoiesis, which explains the higher content of red blood cells in men than in women.

Lecture 29.

<u>Topic: Private physiology of CNS. Functions of the spinal cord.</u>

The goal is to know the functions of the different parts of the spinal cord.

The objectives are.

(a) Reveal the functional feature of neurons in the posterior, anterior, and lateral horns of the spinal cord;

b) indicate the features of phasic, tonic and autonomic reflexes;

c) Bell-Majandie law;

d) the conductive function of the spinal cord.

Content:

The spinal cord is located in the spinal canal and has two main functions: 1) reflex and 2) conductive. All spinal cord reflexes can be divided into: 1) somatic (tonic and phasic) and 2) autonomic. In 1811, Bellah, destroying the anterior spinal roots of the spinal cord of the lumbar segments, noted the loss of motor function of the hind limbs. In 1822 Majandi, destroying the posterior roots of the spinal cord of the lumbar segments, noted loss of sensation of the skin of the lower extremities. Thus, in the posterior roots pass sensitive centripetal nerve fibers from receptors of the skin (pain, temperature, tactile and pressure), muscles, tendons, joints (proprioceptive system) and from receptors of internal organs (autonomic system); in the anterior roots pass motor centrifugal nerve fibers from neurons to muscles. This peculiarity of the function of the posterior and anterior roots of the spinal cord is reflected in the Bell-Majandi law.

Alpha and gamma motoneurons in the anterior horns of the spinal cord are involved in somatic reflexes. The axons of these neurons terminate in extrafusal (alpha motoneurons) and intrafusal (gamma motoneurons) muscles. Phasic reflexes include all antagonistic reflexes (flexion-extension, abduction-adduction, etc.). These reflexes are realized in phases: muscles contract quickly and relax quickly. As a rule, white muscles (type I muscles) are involved in these reflexes. Tonic reflexes are prolonged muscle contractions (Fig.). Red muscles (types IIA and IIB) are involved in these reflexes. Tonic reflexes can be divided into peripheral and central reflexes. Peripheral tonic reflexes are realized by relaxation of extrafusal muscles, which leads to stretching of the nuclear pouch of the muscle spindle (skeletal muscle stretch receptors). This excites the receptors of the nuclear bag, impulses along afferent fibers through the posterior roots of the spinal cord go to the alpha motoneurons of the anterior roots and from here along efferent fibers impulses go to the extrafusal muscles, their contraction occurs. Central tonic reflexes are realized due to the reticulo-spinal pathway. Impulses from the RF brain neurons go to the gamma motoneurons of the anterior roots of the spinal cord, from here along efferent pathways to the intrafusal muscles, during the contraction of which the nuclear bag is stretched. This excites the receptors of the nuclear pouch, impulses along afferent fibers through the posterior roots of the spinal cord go to the alpha motoneurons of the anterior roots and from here along efferent fibers impulses go to the extrafusal muscles, and their contraction occurs (Fig.). Thus, the tension of the nuclear pouch of the muscle spindle (excitation of muscle proprioreceptors) occurs in two ways: 1) by relaxation of extrafusal muscles and 2) by contraction of intrafusal muscles.

Autonomic reflexes are the response of internal organs. These reflexes are realized due to axons of autonomic neurons located in the lateral horns of the spinal cord and constituting the peripheral nerves of the sympathetic and parasympathetic sections of the ANS. These reflexes are involved in the regulation of blood pressure, heart activity, secretion and motor function of the digestive tract and function of the genitourinary system.

Conductive function of the spinal cord. The white matter of the spinal cord includes myelinated nerve fibers that are bundled together to form the conductive pathways of the spinal cord. Short associative fibers provide intersegmental connections. Long projection fibers are divided into ascending, going to different parts of the brain, and descending - from the brain to the spinal cord. Ascending conductive pathways:

1) Tactile sensitivity - sensation of touch and pressure: a) wedge-shaped bundle (Burdach's bundle) from the receptors of the upper body and b/fins: b) thin bundle (Gol's bundle) from the receptors of the lower body and n/fins. Touch receptors include the Meissner cells in the cutaneous papillae and the Merkel discs in the fingertips. The pressure receptors include pachiniev cells in the fascia and tendons. From these receptors impulses go to the posterior roots and on the same side to the medulla oblongata (here the second neuron). Here there is a crossover in the opposite direction to the thalamic nuclei (third neuron) and from here to the cortical end of the analyzer (posterior central gyrus); b) in addition to these pathways, tactile sensitivity is conducted by the ventral spinothalamic pathway. From the tactile receptors to the canalicular interneurons, whose axons pass 2-3 segments along the same side, then pass to the other side and up to the thalamus.

2) The pathway of pain and temperature sensitivity, or the dorsal spinothalamic pathway, is from nociceptors and thermoreceptors to the canalicular interneurons, from here to the opposite side and to the thalamus.

3)	Dorsal cerebrospinal tract (Flexig's bundle) - from receptors of muscles, ligaments and skin of the limbs, without crossing this pathway ends in the cerebellar cortex.

4)	Ventral cerebrospinal tract (Hoovers bundle) - this pathway reaches the cerebellar cortex after crossing over. The Flexig and Hovers bundles transmit information from tendons, skin and visceroreceptors. These pathways are involved in maintaining muscle tone during movement and maintaining body posture in space.

Downstream conductive pathways:

1)	Pyramidal, or corticospinal, which is divided into lateral and anterior fascicles. The lateral bundle starts from the PMA neurons and crosses at the level of the medulla oblongata, descending to the opposite side of the spinal cord. The anterior bundle makes a crossing at the level of the segment in which it terminates. These pathways provide a connection between the motor area neurons of the PMA and the alpha motoneurons of the spinal cord and are responsible for voluntary movements.

2)	The rubrospinal (red-nuclear-spiny cerebellar) tract (Manakova) belongs to the extrapyramidal system, makes a crossing after leaving the red nucleus, connects the neurons of the red nucleus of the midbrain with the cerebellum, medulla oblongata and spinal cord - controls muscle tone and involuntary coordination of movements.

3)	The vestibulospinal also belongs to the extrapyramidal system and is responsible for communication between the Deiters nucleus of the varicose bridge, cerebellum and alpha motoneurons of the anterior horns of the spinal cord. It regulates muscle tone, coordination of movements, balance and orientation in space.

4) Reticulospinal pathway - also belongs to the extrapyramidal system. Depending on in which neurons of the spinal cord this pathway terminates, the following functions are distinguished (Fig.): a) inhibition of spinal reflexes - in this pathway ends on Renshaw cells, their excitation leads to hyperpolarization of alpha motoneurons, which leads to inhibition; b) facilitation of spinal reflexes - in this pathway ends on inhibitory interneurons, their excitation leads to inhibition of Renshaw cells, so the inhibitory effect of these cells on alpha motoneurons is removed, spinal reflexes are facilitated; c) increases the tone of skeletal muscles - in this case the pathway ends at gamma motoneurons of the spinal cord, their excitation leads to contraction of intrafusal muscles, there is a tension of the nuclear bag, excitation of receptors, increased flow of impulses along the afferent pathway through the posterior roots of the spinal cord to alpha motoneurons, the excitation of which increases muscle tone.

Complete crossing of the spinal cord leads to spinal shock. As a result, all types of reflex activity disappear below the transection: motor activity, all types of sensitivity, and autonomic functions are impaired (urination and fecal discharge become involuntary). The cause of shock is mainly due to the loss of communication with the PMA. This is proven by repeated transection of the spinal cord, below the site of transection. In this case, spinal shock does not occur again.

Lecture 30

Topic: Private physiology of the CNS. Functions of the medulla oblongata and midbrain (classification of tonic reflexes according to Magnus)

The goal is to know the functions of the medulla oblongata and midbrain and be able to use this knowledge to understand the functional activities of the CNS.

The objectives are.

(a) Show the role of the medulla oblongata and midbrain in producing tonic reflexes (Magnus classification);

b) point out the main automatic centers in the medulla oblongata;

Content:

The medulla oblongata. Performs two functions: 1) reflex and 2) conductive. Reflex function is carried out due to: a) nuclei of 8 pairs of cranial nerves (VIII-XII); b) automatic centers (respiratory, vasomotor, sneezing, coughing, blinking, vomiting, pyloric); c) participation of medulla oblongata neurons in tonic reflexes (static reflexes). Tonic reflexes provide regulation of muscle tone. Afferent impulses that cause these reflexes come from the vestibular branch of the VIII pair of cranial nerves, the spinal nerves, conducting impulses from the receptors of the muscles of the face, neck, limbs and trunk. All tonic reflexes Magnus divided into two groups: 1) static - when the receptors of this reflex are irritated, they condition a certain position of the body in space; 2) statokinetic - they maintain the balance of the body in space when it moves. Static reflexes in turn can be divided into two groups: 1) posnotonic - provide a certain posture of the body in space; 2) setting, or straightening - provide the return of the body from an unnatural position to a normal one (from a horizontal position to a standing position). The center of static post-tonic reflexes is located in the medulla oblongata, and the center of static erective and statokinetic reflexes is in the midbrain. Afferent pathways of these reflexes begin with receptors of the vestibular apparatus (cochlear vestibule and semicircular tubules), proprioreceptors of the neck muscles and tactile receptors of the skin of the trunk on the side. The importance of neck muscle proprioreceptors: when the head is tilted backward, the tone of the extensor muscles of the upper extremities increases and the tone of the extensor muscles of the lower extremities decreases; when the head is bent toward the rib cage, the tone of the extensor muscles of the upper extremities decreases and the tone of the extensor muscles of the lower extremities increases; when turning the head to the left - the tone of the upper limb extensor muscles on the left increases and the tone of the flexor muscles on the right increases; when turning the head to the right - the tone of the upper limb extensor muscles on the right increases and the tone of the flexor muscles on the left increases. Straightening reflexes are carried out in two phases: 1) lifting of the head - due to irritation of receptors of the vestibular apparatus (vestibule of the cochlea) and skin surface of the trunk; 2) straightening of the trunk - due to irritation of proprioreceptors of the neck muscles and skin surface of the trunk. Statokinetic reflexes are realized during the rotational test - vestibulomotor, vestibulovegetative and vestibulosensory reflexes occur (see vestibular analyzer).

Conductive function of the medulla oblongata - all ascending and descending pathways pass through it

Varolian Bridge - it includes the nuclei of the V-VII cranial nerves, the vestibular nucleus (lateral nucleus of Deiters and upper nucleus of Bekhterev. Facial nerve (VII) innervates facial mimic muscles, hyoid and submandibular salivary, transmits information from the taste buds of the anterior part of the tongue gland. The retractor nerve (VI) innervates the rectus externalis muscle of the eye, which pulls the eyeball outward. The trigeminal nerve (V) - the motor nucleus innervates the masseter muscles, the muscles of the palatine curtain and the muscles that tense the tympanic membrane. The sensitive nucleus receives impulses from receptors of the facial skin, nasal mucosa, teeth, periosteum of the bones of the skull, conjunctiva of the eyeball. The pneumotoxic center, or inhibitory inspiratory neuron (TIN), which triggers the act of exhalation, is located in the varicular bridge. The vestibular nucleus is responsible for the primary analysis of vestibular stimuli.

Midbrain: quadriplegium nuclei, red nucleus, nuclei of the I-IV pairs of cranial nerves, black substance. The anterior tubercles of the quadratochalmia (upper), or optic tubercles carry out reflexes in response to light stimuli (orienting reflex to light stimulus), pupillary reflex, eye accommodation. The posterior tubercles of the quadratochalmia (lower), or auditory - realizes the orienting reflex to sound. The nuclei of the quadratochalmia provide a "watchdog" reflex - preparing the body for a new sudden stimulus. The black substance coordinates swallowing and chewing, contributes to the realization of small movements of the fingers, which require great precision.

Red nucleus. The function of the red nucleus has been studied in decerebrating animals: to dissect the brain between the upper and lower tubercles of the quadratochalmia. In this case, impulses from the red nucleus do not go to the lower parts of the CNS - decerebration rehydration develops (the tone of extensor muscles sharply increases: limbs straighten, head tilts and tail rises. This rehydration can be reduced by destruction of the Deiters nucleus and adjacent neural structures of the reticular formation. Thus, connections of the red nucleus with the spinal cord, the nucleus deuterosus, and the brainstem reticular formation play a major role in the development of decerebratory regidity. When the red nucleus is stimulated via rubrospinal pathways, motoneurons of flexor muscles are excited and motoreurons of extensor muscles are inhibited. When stimulating the nuclei of Deiters and Schwalbe through the vestibulo-spinal tract, there is inhibition of motoneurons of flexor muscles and excitation of motoneurons of extensor muscles. Reticular structures of the medulla oblongata and midbrain have the opposite effect.

Lecture 31.

**<u>Topic: Private physiology of the CNS. Functions of
cerebellum, reticular formation and hypothalamus.</u>**

The goal is to know the functions of the reticular formation of the cerebellum, and hypothalamus and be able to use this knowledge to understand the functional activities of the CNS.

The objectives are.

(a) State the consequences of unilateral and bilateral cerebellar lesions and the main clinical symptoms seen in cerebellar lesions;

b) show the role of reticulo-spinal and reticulo-cortical pathways;

c) point out the main functions of the hypothalamus.

Content:

Reticular formation of the brain - represented by a diffuse cluster of cells of different types and sizes, separated by many multidirectional fibers. This section was so named by Deiters in 1885 for its characteristic cytoarchitectonics. The RF is located in the central part of the brainstem (between the thalamus and the spinal cord). It received the name of reticular formation, or network formation, due to its network connections with almost all CNS structures.

I.M. Sechenov described for the first time the state of spinal reflexes from the state of brain stem structures in 1863, irritating the optic tubercles with sodium chloride crystals and noted the inhibition of spinal reflexes. The works of Megun and his collaborators (1944-1950) showed that when the medial part of the reticular formation is irritated, spinal reflexes are inhibited, and when other RF structures are irritated, these reflexes are facilitated. When the RF structures are irritated through the reticulospinal pathways, the following functions are realized: 1) inhibition of spinal reflexes - in this case impulses arrive to inhibitory Renshaw cells and through them cause hyperpolarization of alpha motoneurons; 2) facilitation of spinal reflexes - in this case impulses arrive to inhibitory interneurons, and through them cause inhibition of Renshaw cells; 3) enhancement of tonic reflexes - in this case impulses arrive to gamma motoneurons, at excitation of which there is a contraction of intrafusal muscles of the muscle spindle, which eventually leads to excitation of alpha motoneurons. Ascending pathways from the RF: 1) reticulocortical pathways - from the center of Magoon Morucia - increases the tone of PMA neurons - awake state; 2) connection with the hypothalamus and limbic system (amygdala complex, hippocampus and cingulate gyrus) - this pathway provides a holistic response of the body and regulates autonomic and homeostatic functions of the body.

The cerebellum performs the function of coordination and regulation of voluntary and involuntary movements. These functions are provided by multiple connections of the cerebellum with the spinal cord and other brain structures: 1) spinocerebellar pathway - informs the cerebellum about the tone of skeletal muscles; 2) a branch from the corticospinal pathway carries information about the necessary tone of skeletal muscles; 3) cerebellospinal pathway - this pathway corrects the necessary tone of skeletal muscles in a particular situation (by comparing signals from the spinocerebellar pathway and corticospinal pathway) 1-3 pathways provide coordination of the body in space during conscious movements; 4) bilateral connection of cerebellum with medulla oblongata and midbrain - this pathway provides coordination of unconscious movements; 5) bilateral connection with hypothalamus and thalamus - provides coordination of sensory and vegetative functions.

The following symptoms are observed in experimental unilateral cerebellar lesions: 1) maneuvering movements - the animal moves in a circle; 2) corkscrew movements - if a frog is lowered into water, it makes corkscrew movements. Both symptoms are associated with the fact that in unilateral cerebellar lesion there is a pronounced dystonia - on the affected side the tone of flexor muscles increases and the tone of extensor muscles disappears, and on the healthy side vice versa: the tone of extensor muscles increases and the tone of flexor muscles disappears. In bilateral lesions there is complete immobility, the animal cannot move independently. In the clinic, a partial cerebellar lesion is noted and the following clinical symptoms are distinguished: the first three symptoms were described by Luciani and named three a, as all symptoms begin with the letter a: 1) asthenia - rapid muscle fatigue, as in this case "extra" muscle groups are involved in the motor act due to the lesion of 1-3 pathways; 2) atonia - lack of tone of skeletal muscles, then it was found that muscle tone does not completely disappear, but there is a disturbance of tone (tone of some muscles increases, others decrease), so it is more correct to call this symptom dystonia; 3) astasia - loss of the ability of muscles to tetanic contraction - this symptom is manifested in the fact that the movement is rocking different parts of the body; in addition to the above symptoms are observed 4) dysarthria - violation of fluency of speech; 5) dysmetria - violation of proportionality of movement, usually in the direction of increase; 6) ataxia - violation of coordination of movement, uncertain gait; 7) equilibrium - violation of balance when walking.

Hypothalamus: gray tubercle, mamillary bodies, and gray matter forming the floor and walls of the 3rd ventricle. The extensive connection of the hypothalamus with the PMA, cerebellum, RF, parasympathetic nuclei of the medulla oblongata, sympathetic nuclei of the spinal cord, thalamus, and pituitary gland provides the diversity of its functions provided by 32 pairs of nuclei, which are subdivided into five groups: 1) nuclei of the preoptic area; 2) anterior group of nuclei; 3) external group of nuclei; 4) middle group of nuclei; 5) posterior group of nuclei. The functions of the hypothalamus include: 1) it is the supreme center of the ANS: the posterior group of nuclei increases the sympathetic tone, and the anterior group of nuclei increases the parasympathetic tone (see ANS section). These nuclei take part in the formation of the autonomic component of emotions; 2) the highest center of endocrine function - through the system of liberins and statins it regulates the production of tropic hormones, which in turn regulate the production of effector hormones through the endocrine glands (see endocrine physiology section). Liberins and statins are involved in the formation of the endocrine component of emotion; 3) participates in thermoregulation through the thermoregulation center, which consists of two divisions - the center of heat dissipation and the center of heat production (see the functional system that ensures the constancy of body temperature); 4) participates in the regulation of sleep and wakefulness. The Hess center is found here, the excitation of which causes inhibition of the awake center of Morucia Magoon, which leads to the spilt inhibition of the PMA - the emergence of sleep; 5) participates in the regulation of digestion and the formation of food motivation (see physiology of digestion): irritation of the external nuclei (hunger center) causes the sensation of hunger, irritation of the ventromedial nuclei (satiety center) causes the refusal of food; 6) due to osmoreceptors regulates the osmotic pressure of blood through the change of diuresis (see physiology of kidneys); 7) participates in the regulation of digestion and the formation of food motivation (see physiology of kidneys). physiology of kidneys); 7) due to effector hormones vasopressin (antidiuretic) and oxytocin it participates in the regulation of diuresis, BP (vasopressin), uterine contractions and muscles of mammary gland alveoli (oxytocin); 8) it is a part of CNS, participating in the formation of emotions (see physiology of emotions); 9) it participates in adaptive behavior through various biological motivations (see physiology of biological motivations). The hypothalamus is the peutzmecker of all biological motivations.

Lecture 32.

**Topic: I.P. Pavlov's doctrine of analyzers. Characteristics of
the visual analyzer.**

Purpose - to know the functional organization of the analyzers, their importance; optical characteristics and regulation of the dioptric apparatus of the eye, its receptor apparatus.

The objectives are.

(a) Specify the constituent parts of the analyzer and their features;

b) show the photochemical processes occurring in the retina;

c) reveal theories of color vision;

d) give the physiological mechanisms of accommodation, types of disorder and their causes;

Content:

Analyzer - this term was introduced by I.P. Pavlov in 1909 to designate a set of formations providing perception and analysis of information about the external and internal environment of the organism and forming specific sensations. Any analyzer consists of three components: 1) peripheral part - receptors; 2) conductive part; 3) cortical part. Receptor is a specialized structure, which in the process of evolution has adapted to the perception of the appropriate stimulus of the external or internal world. Any receptor performs the following functions: 1) perceives the action of the stimulus; 2) converts (encodes) the energy of the stimulus into a nerve impulse; 3) primitive analysis (signal differentiation) takes place in receptors, as evidenced by the presence of specific receptors (photoreceptors, phonoreceptors, baroreceptors, etc.). Each receptor is able to distinguish from a multitude of stimuli only the adequate, i.e. corresponding to the given receptor. The conductive part of the analyzer contributes to the conduction of the transformed signal from

125

the receptors to the cortical part. The following features are distinguished: 1) multichannel conduction of the same information, which ensures the reliability of impulse transmission; 2) multilevel conduction of excitation due to multiple switching (in ganglia, spinal cord, reticular formation, thalamus), which ensures higher analysis of the signal according to its various parameters; 3) unification of signals (for example, in the reticular formation of the brain), which ensures the interaction of the signal with the cortical part of the analyzer. The cortical part of the analyzer provides the emergence of certain sensations corresponding to each analyzer and perception. Sensations are a subjective image of the objectively existing world, it is a reflection of the properties of the objects of the objective world. Perception is the interpretation of sensations in accordance with one's experience, i.e. recognition of the image. The following structural and functional zones are distinguished: 1) primary projection zone - located in layer IV, in this zone the formation of sensations, conscious and subconscious perception of stimuli action takes place; 2) secondary projection zone, here the interaction of analyzers and more complex processing of information takes place; 3) tertiary zone - associative cortex, here the further processing of information takes place with its use for the formation of psychophysiological processes (perception, emotions, thinking).

The visual analyzer is a set of formations that ensures the perception of electromagnetic radiation with wavelengths of the visible range (400-700 nm) and the formation of light sensations. 90% of information about the external environment is provided by the visual analyzer. The peripheral part of this analyzer is represented by the dioptric apparatus of the eye and the retina. The dioptric apparatus forms an inverted and reduced image of the external world on the retina and is represented by the following components: cornea, fluid chambers, iris, pupil, lens and its bag, vitreous body, lacrimal gland secretion. The refractive power of the cornea and anterior chamber is 43D, of the flattened lens is 19.1D, of the whole eye is 58.6D. Retina is a part of the intermediate brain, brought to the periphery, has the following layers: 1) pigment layer of melanin-containing epithelial cells, absorbs light, is involved in the trophic receptors (depot vit. A), the weakest place (depot vit. A). A), the weakest place (retinal detachment); 2) layer of photoreceptors; 3) layer of horizontal cells (inhibitory neurons); 4) layer of bipolar cells; 5) layer of bipolar cells (inhibitory neurons); 6) layer of ganglion cells (occurrence of PD, formation of optic nerve). Photoreceptors of the eye - rods and three types of cones: 1) rods (about 120 million) are located in the retina except for the yellow and blind spots and perform the following functions: have high sensitivity to light (500 times higher than cones) and are adapted for night vision; provide peripheral vision; perceive moving objects; 2) cones (about 6 million) are located in the yellow spot and central fossa, in this area visual acuity is maximum, provide central vision, visual acuity and color perception.

Color vision - is carried out by cones. The three-component theory of color vision (T. Jung, 1802; G. Helmholtz, 1859) assumes the presence of three types of cones: 1) cones with visual pigment absorbing electromagnetic waves of 420 nm (blue color); 2) cones with visual pigment absorbing electromagnetic waves of 530 nm (green color); 3) cones with visual pigment absorbing electromagnetic waves of 560 nm (red color). Different colors are formed as a result of unequal stimulation of each cone (white color due to equal stimulation of all types of cones; equal stimulation of red and green cones gives the perception of yellow color). Violation of color perception (congenital forms of color blindness - old name - color blindness) is due to the lack of genes encoding different types of opsin in cones (red and green opsin genes are located in the X chromosome, blue opsin gene - in the 7th chromosome). A distinction is made between: 1) dichromasia (absence of perception of one color): a) deuteranopia (6%) - absence of opsin perceiving green color (green-blind); b) protanopia (1.1%) - absence of opsin perceiving red color (red-blind); c) tritanopia (0.01%) - absence of opsin perceiving blue color (blue-blind); 2) achromasia (less than 0.01% - complete color blindness (black and white perception).

Accomodation of the eye. Accommodation disorder. Eye accommodation is the ability of the eye to see both distant objects and close objects clearly. The mechanism of accommodation of the eye is due to two factors: 1) the elasticity of the lens, due to which the convexity of the lens can vary from 19D to 33D. With age, the elasticity of the crystalline lens decreases and reaches its minimum after 60 years of age, resulting in senile hyperopia - presbyopia; 2) the accommodative muscle, or ciliary muscle (page 66, Fig. Zh2, Zh3): a) when the accommodative muscle is contracted (p. 66, Fig. Zh2), the cine ligaments are relaxed and due to the elasticity of the lens, it becomes more convex, the refractive power of the eye increases and such an eye sees close objects clearly; b) when the accommodative muscle is relaxed (p. 66, Fig. Zh3), the cine ligaments are relaxed (p. 66, Fig. Zh3), the eye sees close objects clearly. 66, Fig.Zh3) the cine ligaments are stretched and due to the elasticity of the crystalline lens its convexity decreases (lens flattening occurs), the refractive power of the eye decreases and such an eye sees distant objects clearly. The most common types of accommodation disorders are myopia (nearsightedness) and hypermetropia (farsightedness). To detect these types of accommodation disorder it is necessary to completely relax the accommodative muscle, which is done by injecting atropine solution into the eye. In a normal eye (emmetropic eye), the retina coincides with the main focal length of the optical system of the eye, so there is a clear vision of the object. In the myopic eye, as a result of the elongated anatomical axis, the main focal length is in front of the retina, so there is a blurred image. In the hyperopic eye, as a result of the short anatomical axis, the principal focal length is behind the retina, so a blurred image is noted. Thus, in myopic and hyperopic eyes at full relaxation of the accommodative muscle the same result is observed - blurred image on the retina. The reason for this is different: in myopic eye the blurred image on the retina occurs due to the fact that the main focus of the myopic eye is in front of the retina, closer to the retina (myopia); in hyperopic eye - due to the fact that the main focus of the eye is behind the retina, further from the retina (hyperopia). Correction of myopic eye is performed by reducing the optical system of the eye (its refractive power), as the main focus is in front of the retina - this is achieved with the help of double-curved (diffusing) lenses.

Correction of hyperopic eyes is performed by increasing the optical system of the eye (its refractive power), as the main focus is behind the retina - this is achieved by using double-convex (collecting) lenses. It should be noted that weak myopia is self-correctable due to tension (contraction of the accommodative muscle) of accommodation, as this type of disorder was determined with complete relaxation of the accommodative muscle. Mild hyperopia cannot be self-corrected, because for correction it is necessary to relax the accommodative muscle, and this type of accommodation disorder was detected with full relaxation of the accommodative muscle.

Lecture 33.

Topic: I.P. Pavlov's doctrine of analyzers. Characteristics of auditory and vestibular analyzers.

Objective - structural and functional characterization of the auditory and vestibular analyzers.

The objectives are.

(a) Disclose sound-capturing, sound-conducting, and sound-receiving apparatuses;

b) give theories of the perception of sounds of different frequencies;

c) indicate the occurrence of reflexes arising from irritation of receptors of the vestibular analyzer.

Content:

Hearing organ - consists of the outer, middle and inner ear. The outer ear is represented by the auricle and the external ear canal. The middle ear is represented by three interconnected auditory ossicles: the malleus, incus, and stapes. The malleus is attached to the tympanic membrane and the stapes to the oval window. The auditory ossicles amplify sound 20 times. The middle ear cavity communicates with the nasopharynx by means of the eustachian (auditory) tube, so that the air pressure in the middle ear cavity is maintained at atmospheric pressure. The auditory tube opens during swallowing. The middle ear is separated from the outer ear by the tympanic membrane, which is 9 mm in diameter. The inner ear is represented by the vestibule (uterus, sac), the three semicircular tubules and the cochlea (tympanic and vestibular ladders). The cochlear vestibule and semicircular tubules belong to the vestibular analyzer and the cochlea to the auditory analyzer. The preauricular cavity, tympanic and vestibular ladders of the cochlea are filled with perilymph, while the semicircular canals, rete, sac and the cochlear duct (the membranous canal of the cochlea) located in the perilymph are filled with endolymph. There is an electrical potential (intracochlear, or endocochlear potential) of about +80 mV between the endolymph and perilymph. The hair cells of the cortical organ are polarized by the endocochlear potential to a critical level, which increases their sensitivity to mechanical action. Endolymph is a viscous fluid formed by the vascular band of the cochlear canal and fills the membranous canal of the cochlea and connects with the endolymph of the vestibular apparatus through a special channel (duktus reuniens). The concentration of potassium ions in the endolymph is 100 times higher and the concentration of sodium ions is 10 times lower than in the perilymph. Perilymph is chemically similar to blood plasma and liquor and occupies an intermediate position between them in terms of protein content.

Auditory analyzer - provides perception of sound vibrations with frequency from 16-20 Hz to 16-20 kHz and formation of sound sensations. The receptor part of the auditory analyzer - the spiral (cortical) organ is located in the cochlea. The basilar (main) and vestibular membranes located inside the cochlea divide the canal cavity into three parts: the tympanic ladder, the vestibular ladder, and the membranous canal of the cochlea (middle ladder). Endolymph fills the cochlear membranous canal, and perilymph fills the vestibular and tympanic staircases. In the membranous canal of the cochlea, the cochlear receptor apparatus, the corticoid organ, containing several rows of cells (supporting and hair cells), is located on the base membrane. All cells are attached to the main membrane, and hair cells are connected with the covering membrane by their free surface. The path of sound vibrations to hair cells is as follows: sound - auricle - external auditory canal - tympanic membrane - malleus - anvil - stirrup - oval window membrane - perilymph (at the transition of sound from air to liquid there is a sharp decrease in energy and amplitude of sound, sound pressure increases (2 times) and sound speed increases (4 times), the frequency of sound does not change) - basilar and tectoral membranes - round window membrane. The fluid displaced by the displacement of the oval window membrane creates excess pressure in the vestibular canal. Under the action of this pressure, the basement membrane shifts towards the tympanic ladder, which leads to displacement of the tectorial membrane relative to the hair cells, their excitation occurs (depolarization of the hair cell membrane). In the synapses between the receptor cell and afferent nerve ending, the neurotransmitter - glutamate - is released, causes depolarization of the postsynaptic membrane and PD generation occurs. High frequency sound waves travel a short distance along the basilar membrane; medium frequency sound waves travel about half way and then stop; low frequency sound waves travel along the membrane almost to the helicotreme (apex of the cochlea). Conductive section of the auditory analyzer: afferent nerve fibers from the cochlea enter the spiral ganglion and from it enter the dorsal (posterior) and ventral (anterior) cochlear nuclei, located in the upper part of the medulla oblongata. From here ascending nerve fibers form synapses with second-order neurons, the axons of which partly pass to the opposite side to the nuclei of the upper olive, and partly end on the nuclei of the upper olive of the same side. From the nuclei of the upper olive auditory pathways as part of the lateral lemniscus pathway, some fibers end in the lateral lemniscus nuclei, and most of the axons bypass these nuclei and follow to the lower bicolumn, where they form synapses. From here the auditory pathway passes to the medial patellar bodies and from here to the superior gyrus of the temporal lobe of the cerebral cortex. The cortical section of the auditory analyzer is represented by: 1) primary auditory cortex - 41st field, Heschl's gyrus of the temporal lobe deep in the sylvian sulcus and 42nd field of the superior temporal gyrus - forms the sense of tones, noises, sounds; 2) secondary auditory cortex - 22nd field of the superior temporal gyrus of the left hemisphere - forms the understanding of the sequence of sounds, words; 22nd field of the right hemisphere - understanding of the sequence of tones (melody), intonation, gender of the voice.

The perception of sounds of different frequencies is explained by Bekeshi's hydrodynamic theory. When low frequency sounds are perceived, the entire perilymph from the base of the cochlea to the apex oscillates (Fig. Zh10), which leads to bending of the main membrane at the apex of the cochlea and excitation of receptors of the Cortium organ in the apex region, which leads to excitation of the corresponding cells in the PMA. During perception of high frequency sounds, a small column oscillation occurs, which leads to bending of the main membrane at the base of the cochlea and excitation of receptors of the Cortium organ also at the base of the cochlea, which leads to excitation of other cells in the PMA.

The vestibular analyzer is a set of formations that provide spatial orientation of the body at rest and in motion. It perceives information about the position, linear and angular movements of the body and head. Receptors of this analyzer are located in the three semicircular tubules and the vestibule of the cochlea. The vestibule consists of two sections: the saccule (sacculus) and the utricle (utriculus). In these sections there are small elevations - maculae (spots), which contain the otolithic apparatus - a cluster of receptor cells, which are covered with a jelly-like mass consisting of mucopolysaccharides. Due to the presence of calcium phosphorus-carbon dioxide crystals in it, it is called otolith membrane. An adequate stimulus to the otolith apparatus is straight-line motion, acceleration or deceleration, head and body inclinations, as well as rocking and shaking. In the semicircular tubules, the jelly-like mass does not contain otoliths and is called the cupula. The adequate stimulus to the receptors of the semicircular tubules (hair tassels) is rotary movements. The first conductance neuron are bipolar cells located in the vestibular ganglion. The peripheral outgrowths of these neurons contact the receptors, and the central ones as part of the vestibular nerve (VIII pair of cranial nerves) are directed to the vestibular nuclei of the medulla oblongata - the second neuron (Deiters, Bekhterev, Schwalbe, Roller). From here the impulses go to different parts of the CNS: thalamic nuclei, cerebellum, nuclei of the oculomotor nerve, motoneurons of the cervical spinal cord, reticular formation, hypothalamus. Due to the above-mentioned connections the following reflexes are realized at irritation of receptors of the vestibular analyzer: 1) vestibulomotor reflexes: a) due to changes in the tone of the muscles of the eye there is eye nystagmus - slow eye movement towards rotation with a quick return to the initial state; b) due to changes in the tone of the muscles of the neck and head - head nystagmus - slow head movement towards rotation with a quick return to the initial state; c) due to changes in the tone of the muscles of the trunk and limbs (via vestibulo-, reticulo- and rubrospinal pathways) - deviation of the body towards rotation during rectilinear movement after rotation. This occurs due to the fact that on the side of rotation the tone of flexor muscles increases, and on the opposite side - the tone of extensor muscles; 2) vestibulovegetative reflexes - changes in the work of internal organs after the rotational test due to the connection of vestibular nuclei with the hypothalamus; 3) vestibulosensory reflexes - changes in the sensitivity threshold of receptors of other analyzers.

Lecture 34.

Topic: The pain analyzer. Current understanding of nociception and central mechanisms of pain. Antinociceptive system. Neurochemical mechanisms of antinociception.

Objective - to know the physiological characteristics of the pain analyzer, its receptor, conductive and cortical compartments.

The objectives are.

(a) To reveal the biological significance of pain and the modern concept of nociception;

b) show the theories and central mechanisms of pain;

c) give the role of cortex, subcortical formations and humoral factors in the formation of the response to nociceptive stimuli;

d) specify the principles of classification of analgesics.

Content:

The pain or nociceptive analyzer is a set of formations that form the sensation of pain under physical and chemical influences that have a damaging effect on the body. The difference between pain and other sensations is that it does not inform the brain about the quality of the stimulus, but indicates that the stimulus is damaging. Components of pain: 1) sensory - pain as a sensation; 2) affective - emotional, autonomic and motor manifestations of pain; 3) need-motivational - pain as a negative biological need that forms pain control behavior; 4) cognitive - evaluation of pain sensations, formed in the frontal cortex. Theories of pain: 1) theory of intensity (E. Darwin, 1794; A. Goldscheider, 1886) - according to this theory there are no specific pain receptors, pain occurs at irritation of any receptors at the action of supermaximal stimuli; 2) theory of specificity (M. Frey, 1894) - suggests the presence of specific receptors (nociceptors), irritation of which occurs at the action of damaging stimuli (nocio -

damaging); 3) theory of gates (R. Melzack, 1973), according to this theory, pain occurs at irritation of any receptors at the action of damaging stimuli. Melzack, 1973), according to this theory, pain sensations arise from the inhibition of special neurons of the gelatinous substance (a cluster of neurons located in the 2nd and 3rd plates according to Rexed), due to which impulses from nociceptors along the spinothalamic pathway reach the central structures of this analyzer. Excitation of gelatinous substance neurons causes inhibition of neurons of spinothalamic pathways, and pain sensations cease. The activity of neurons of the gelatinous substance is maintained in 3 ways, which are included in the antinociceptive system. Inhibition of gelatinous substance neurons occurs when nociceptors are irritated. Pain receptors (nociceptors) are free endings of sensitive myelinated and unmyelinated nerve fibers, which are localized in the skin, mucous membranes, periosteum, teeth, muscles, organs of thoracic and abdominal cavities (the density of nociceptors in the skin is 200 per 1 sq.cm, and on the border of dentin and enamel of the tooth - 7500). Irritants of pain receptors: mechanical (squeezing, stretching, bending, twisting), thermal (thermal, when the temperature exceeds 45 degrees, cold, when the temperature is below 15 degrees), chemical (potassium and hydrogen cations, serotonin, histamine, bradykinin, ADP). The conductive compartment is represented by the spinothalamic pathway: 1) the neospinothalamic pathway (this pathway is absent in lower animals) at the brainstem level conducts pain signals through a specific pathway (spinal cord loop) to specific sensory nuclei of the thalamus. Excitation transmission in the synapses of this pathway is carried out with the help of a fast-acting mediator - glutamate. From specific thalamic nuclei, signals are transmitted to the somatosensory cortex SI and SII. These features form the conduction of "fast" pain and its perception with good localization and characterization of painful stimuli; 2) the paleospinothalamic pathway conducts pain signals through a nonspecific pathway. From nonspecific nuclei of the thalamus impulses arrive not only to the somatosensory cortex, but also to other departments. The transmission of excitation along this pathway is slow, the mediator in the synapses of this pathway is P substance. This pathway is used for "late", poorly localized pain.

The cortical section of the pain analyzer is located in the somatosensory cortex - projection fields SI and SII. The primary SI field provides perception of "fast" pain, with determination of its location on the body. This field is located next to the motor cortex of the anterior central gyrus, due to which the motor defense reaction to the action of a painful stimulus is urgently activated. The inability to clearly define the localization of "slow" pain is explained by the fact that impulses from nonspecific thalamic nuclei arrive not only in the SI and SII fields, but also in other cortical fields. The somatosensory field SII, has a less clear topographic projection of the body. The neurons of this field have stronger bilateral connections with the thalamic nuclei. In addition to the SI and SII fields, the following plays an important role in pain perception: 1) frontal cortex - provides self-assessment of pain (its cognitive component) and forms purposeful pain behavior. In case of lobotomy (cutting the connections between the frontal cortex and thalamus retains the sensation of pain, but it does not bother them (pain does not cause suffering); 2) limbic system (cingulate gyrus, hippocampus, dentate gyrus, amygdala complex of the temporal lobe), contributes to the formation of the emotional component of pain, autonomic, somatic and behavioral reactions.

The antinociceptive system is a set of interrelated structures that reduces the perception of pain sensations. According to Kalyuzhny L.V. (1984) any stimulus that does not cause damage to the body also causes activation of the antinociceptive system, there is a release of a certain portion of opioid peptides that cause euphoria. The antinociceptive system is a reward system, it encourages the body's exploratory activity to actively encounter any stimuli. This system includes: 1) opioid peptides - it is now known that opium and its preparations act on special protein receptors and block the conduction of pain impulses, which contributes to the reduction or disappearance of pain sensations. For these receptors there are endogenous stimulants - opioid peptides - which are products of proteolysis of large inactive precursor peptides formed in the brain, adenohypophysis, cerebral layer of the adrenal glands, gastrointestinal tract, and placenta. Three opioid peptides are currently known: a) endorphins, which are formed from propiomelanocortin; b) enkephalins, formed from proenkephalin A; c) dynorphins, formed from proenkephalin B. They act on three types of opiate receptors: mu (predominantly endorphins), delta (enkephalins), and kappa (dynorphins). Opioids, interacting with their receptors, exert their effects either on the neurons of the gelatinous substance (excite them) or block the transmission of nociceptive impulses. The density of mu and kappa receptors is highest in the cerebral cortex and spinal cord, average density in the brainstem; the density of delta receptors is average in the cerebral cortex and spinal cord, low in the brainstem; 2) the same analgesic action has: a) neurotensin-polypeptide, which is synthesized in various structures of the CNS; b) oxytocin and vasopressin (ADH); c) serotonin - inhibit nociceptive impulsation in the area of the medulla oblongata; d) catecholamines of the cerebral layer of the adrenal glands, which is accompanied by an increase in the secretion of endorphins; e) corticoliberin increases the formation of endorphins in the adenohypophysis and its secretion into the blood; 3) due to impulses coming from mechanoreceptors of the skin, which increase the activity of neurons of the gelatinous substance, which leads to inhibition of neurons of the spinal thalamic pathways; 4) due to impulses of supraspinal structures (frontal lobe, caudate nucleus, thalamic nuclei, cerebellar neurons, hypothalamic centers, red nucleus, black substance, structures of the medulla oblongata), which increase the activity of neurons of the gelatinous substance.

Classification of analgesics depends on the stages of formation of pain sensations. According to this principle, all existing anesthetic agents can be divided into the following groups: 1) local anesthesia - blocks nociceptors in the area of injury; 2) conductive anesthesia blocks nerves conducting impulses from the source of injury to afferent neurons of the spinal cord; 3) epidural anesthesia - blocks spinal nerves at the level of posterior roots of the spinal cord; 4) subarachnoid, or spinal anesthesia - blocks the spinothalamic tract; 5) central analgesia - blocks the activity of CNS structures responsible for the conduction of pain impulses, or enhancing the activity of their own antinociceptive systems; 6) anesthesia, or general anesthesia - blocks PMA neurons that perceive impulses from nociceptors.

Lecture 35.

Topic: Processes occurring in the PMA, their properties. Types of GND according to I.P. Pavlov and Eysenck. Conditioned reflexes and mechanisms of their formation. The concept of dynamic stereotype.

Purpose - to know the concept of GND, the role of conditioned reflex as a form of human adaptation to changing conditions of existence, regularities of formation of conditioned reflexes, the role of dynamic stereotype in learning and acquisition of labor skills, types of GND and their classification.

The objectives are.

(a) Define conditioned reflexes and reveal the mechanisms of their formation;

b) show the difference between conditioned and unconditional reflexes;

c) specify ways of developing conditioned reflexes of different orders;

d) reveal the features of dynamic stereotype and its role in learning and acquisition of labor skills, types of GND and their classification;

e) indicate the peculiarities of PND types according to I.P. Pavlov and Eysenck;

(e) Give the Hippocratic correlation between types of GND and temperament.

Content:

Types of GND is a set of properties of nervous processes occurring in the cortex of the large hemispheres. There are two processes in the cortex - excitation and inhibition. Studying these processes, I.P. Pavlov singled out three properties for each process: 1) strength is estimated by the limit of working capacity of cortical cells and the development of pessimal inhibition. According to this property, strong and weak types are distinguished; 2) equilibrium is determined by the ratio of the strength of excitatory and inhibitory processes. According to this property distinguish balanced and unbalanced types; 3) mobility of nervous processes is determined by the speed (speed) of the change of excitation inhibition and vice versa. According to this property, the mobile and inert types are distinguished.

According to the totality of the three properties, 4 types of GND are distinguished:

1) strong, mobile, unbalanced with predominance of excitation processes ("unrestrained" type);

2) strong, agile, balanced ("lively" type);

3) strong, sedentary (inert), balanced ("calm" or "inert" type);

4) weak - all properties are weakly expressed ("greenhouse"), indecisive, ready to react to a wide range of insignificant signals. A brief characterization of PND types according to I.P. Pavlov can be presented as follows: in the cortex of the large hemispheres (HPA) there are two processes - excitation and inhibition. Each of these processes is characterized by three properties: strength, mobility (speed of change of excitation process by inhibition and vice versa), equilibrium (determined by the correspondence of the strength of excitatory and inhibitory processes). For each property separately, all people are divided into two types: by strength - strong and weak; by mobility - mobile and sedentary (inert); by equilibrium - balanced and unbalanced (unrestrained). According to the totality of the three properties, all people can be divided into four types of GND. The first type is strong, mobile and balanced, or lively. The second type is strong, mobile and unbalanced, or unrestrained.

The third type is strong, little agile and balanced, or inert. The fourth type is weak.

Correspondence of types of VND on IP Pavlov temperaments on Hippocrates: 1 type corresponds to choleric, 2 type - sanguine, 3 type - phlegmatic and 4 type - melancholic.

Types of GNI can be determined using the Eysenck test, which uses 57 statements:

This scheme reflects the method of determining extraversion-introversion according to Eysenck, types of GND according to I.P. Pavlov and temperaments according to Hippocrates. The abscissa axis reflects the degree of expression of extraversion: the number of points from 0 to 11 - these are introverts; from 13 to 24 - these are extroverts. The ordinate axis reflects the degree of neuroticism (stability of nervous processes in the cortex of the large hemispheres): the number of points from 0 to 11 - with stable nervous processes; from 13 to 24 - with unstable nervous processes. The Eysenck scale of extraversion-introversion reflects the property of mobility of nervous processes according to I.P. Pavlov. The Eysenck scale of neuroticism reflects the property of balance of nervous processes according to I.P. Pavlov. The right lower square indicates a stable extrovert (sanguine according to Hippocrates, strong mobile, balanced type according to I.P. Pavlov). The right upper square indicates an unstable extrovert (choleric according to Hippocrates, strong mobile, unbalanced type according to I.P. Pavlov). The left bottom square testifies to a stable introvert (phlegmatic according to Hippocrates, strong sedentary, balanced type according to I.P. Pavlov). The left upper square indicates an unstable introvert (melancholic according to Hippocrates, weak type according to I.P. Pavlov).

24 statements characterizing extraversion- introversion, i.e. by analysis of these statements it is possible to estimate mobility of nervous processes. This scale distinguishes between extroverts (mobile) and introverts (weakly expressed mobility, inertness); 24 statements (neuroticism scale) characterizing stability of nervous processes (equilibrium). This scale distinguishes between people with stable and unstable nervous processes; 9 statements characterize falsity, they determine the degree of readiness of the test subject for testing. Thus, according to two scales (extraversion-introversion and neuroticism) of Eysenck's test we can distinguish 4 types: 1) unstable extrovert (type 1 according to I.P. Pavlov, choleric according to Hippocrates); 2) stable extrovert (type 2 according to I.P. Pavlov, sanguine according to Hippocrates); 3) stable introvert (type 3 according to I.P. Pavlov, phlegmatic according to Hippocrates) and 4) unstable introvert (type 4 according to I.P. Pavlov, melancholic according to Hippocrates). Correspondence of I.P. Pavlov's PND types, Hippocratic temperaments and extraversion-introversion expression is reflected in the following table:

Типы Св-ва		I	II	III	IV
П А В Л О В	С	+	+	+	−
	П	+	+	−	−
	У	+	−	+	−
АЙЗЕНК — Э — э		+	+	−	−
АЙЗЕНК — Э — и		−	−	+	+
АЙЗЕНК — Н — с		+	−	+	−
АЙЗЕНК — Н — нс		−	+	−	+
ГИПОКРАТ		С	Х	Ф	М

This table shows the interaction of types of GND according to Pavlov, extraversion-introversion according to Eysenck and temperaments according to Hippocrates. Hippocrates distinguished four temperaments by the ratio of different body fluids: sanguine (Sa), choleric (X), phlegmatic (F) and melancholic (M). I.P. Pavlov distinguished four types of GND by the properties of excitation and inhibition processes in the PMA. I.P. Pavlov distinguished three properties: strength of excitatory and inhibitory processes (S), mobility (M) and equilibrium of these processes (E). As can be seen from the table, the first type (I) is strong, mobile and balanced, or calm; the second type (II) is strong, mobile, but unbalanced with the predominance of excitation processes, or unrestrained; the third type (III) is strong sedentary and balanced, or inert; the fourth type (IV) is weak, that is, all properties are weakly expressed. Eysenck has allocated two properties for characterization of types of people: 1) expression of extraversion-introversion (E) on which all people can be divided into extroverts and introverts; 2) neuroticism (N), i.e. stability of nervous processes on which all people can be divided into stable and unstable. According to the totality of these properties all people can be divided into four types: 1) stable extrovert; 2) unstable extrovert; 3) stable introvert; 4) unstable introvert. The table shows that extroversion- introversion according to Eysenck corresponds to the mobility of nervous processes according to I.P. Pavlov, and neuroticism according to Eysenck corresponds to the equilibrium of nervous processes according to I.P. Pavlov. Thus, the first type according to I.P. Pavlov is a sanguine according to Hippocrates, or a stable extrovert according to Eysenck; the second type according to I.P. Pavlov is a choleric according to Hippocrates, or an unstable extrovert according to Eysenck; the third type according to I.P. Pavlov is a sanguine according to I.P. Pavlov.The third type according to I.P. Pavlov is phlegmatic according to Hippocrates, or stable introvert according to Eysenck; the fourth type according to I.P. Pavlov is melancholic according to Hippocrates, or unstable introvert according to Eysenck.

Conditioned-reflex activity of the PMA. Inhibition of GND

Conditioned reflex - 1) is a synthesis of two or more unconditional reflexes (Asratyan). The following follows from this definition: a) any conditioned reflex is produced on the basis of an unconditional one (as many unconditional reflexes exist, so many conditioned reflexes can be produced); b) the simultaneous action of two or more stimuli is necessary for the formation of a conditioned reflex; 2) it is an acquired, individual, temporary response to an indifferent (conditioned, inadequate) stimulus with obligatory participation of the cortex of the large hemispheres; 3) these are reactions arising under certain conditions. The main differences between conditioned and unconditional reflexes are: 1) unconditional reflexes are innate (hereditary), that is, these reflexes are genetically predetermined, and conditional reflexes are acquired - they arise if the conditions for their occurrence are met; 2) by prevalence - unconditional reflexes are species-specific, characteristic of the entire species, and conditional reflexes are individual, arise only in those in whom the conditions for their occurrence were met; 3) permanence - unconditional reflexes are permanent, while conditioned reflexes are temporary, they disappear if the conditions for their occurrence are not observed for a long time; 4) stimulus - unconditional reflexes arise to adequate (unconditional, significant) stimuli, while conditioned reflexes arise to inadequate (conditional, insignificant) stimuli; 5) on participation of CNS departments - unconditional reflexes arise with participation of lower and higher CNS departments, and conditioned reflexes - with obligatory participation of the cortex of the large hemispheres (higher CNS departments). Conditions necessary for the development of a conditioned reflex: 1) reinforcement, i.e. for the formation of a conditioned reflex it is necessary to reinforce the action of a conditioned (inadequate) stimulus with the action of an unconditioned (adequate) stimulus. When an isolated conditioned stimulus is used, there is no reaction. In case of simultaneous action of conditioned and unconditioned stimuli (reinforcement), a reaction occurs. The appearance of a reaction to an isolated conditioned stimulus after repeated reinforcement (7-10 times) indicates the formation of a conditioned reflex. According to the type of reinforcement distinguish conditioned reflexes of the first order (reinforcement of a conditioned signal by the action of an unconditional stimulus), conditioned reflexes of the second and higher (in humans 6-7) orders. When developing a conditioned reflex of the second order, a new conditioned signal is used, the action of which is reinforced by a conditioned stimulus (in this case, it acts as an unconditional stimulus) when developing a conditioned reflex of the first order. When developing a conditioned reflex of the third order, a new conditioned signal is used, the action of which is reinforced by a conditioned stimulus (in this case, it plays the role of an unconditional stimulus) when developing a conditioned reflex of the second order, etc.; 2) reinforcement requires anticipation of the action of a conditioned stimulus, i.e., for the formation of a conditioned reflex, the conditioned stimulus is acted upon first, followed by an unconditional stimulus; 3) the strength of a conditioned stimulus should be weaker than the strength of an unconditional stimulus; 4) the active state of the cortex of the large hemispheres, the state of the unconditioned stimulus, and the conditioned stimulus should be weaker than the unconditioned stimulus. Mechanism of the emergence of a conditioned reflex: 1) according to I.P. Pavlov. According to E. Asratyan's definition, a conditioned reflex is a synthesis of two or more unconditional reflexes. From this definition follows: 1) a conditioned reflex is carried out with the obligatory participation of the cortex of the large hemispheres - the PMA (synthesis is carried out in the PMA); 2) any conditioned reflex is carried out on the basis of an unconditioned reflex, so any unconditioned reflex can be conditioned. On the basis of two unconditional reflexes (blinking, salivary secretion), two conditioned reflexes (blinking and salivary secretion) can be developed. The blinking unconditioned reflex is realized by the action of a strong light stimulus. Blinking conditioned reflex is carried out on a weak food stimulus. Unconditional salivary reflex is carried out to a strong food stimulus, and the conditional salivary reflex - to a weak light stimulus. Let's consider the mechanism of occurrence of the conditioned salivary reflex. For this purpose, we conduct reinforcement in the following way: after a weak light stimulus, we act with a strong food stimulus. In this case, two centers of excitation (weak and strong excitation) appear simultaneously in the PMA. According to the principle of dominance, the weak excitation spreads towards the strong one. With repeated reinforcement, a temporary connection between the two centers appears in the cortex of the large hemispheres. The formation of a temporary connection is evidenced by the presence of salivation on the isolated action of a weak light conditioned stimulus. In this case, the light stimulus causes excitation in the PMA, which spreads through a temporary connection to the center that perceives the food stimulus, from here impulses arrive to the salivary glands and salivary reflex occurs.

Thus, during reinforcement in the cortex of the large hemispheres there are two foci of excitation (the center perceiving the conditioned stimulus and the center perceiving the unconditioned stimulus), one of which is dominant (the center perceiving the unconditioned stimulus, because its strength was greater than the strength of the conditioned stimulus), the phenomenon of path retracing is formed due to the transition of excitation from the center perceiving the conditioned stimulus to the center perceiving the unconditioned stimulus. As a result of repeated reinforcement, a temporary connection is formed between the center perceiving the conditioned stimulus and the center perceiving the unconditioned stimulus. The formation of a temporary connection is evidenced by the isolated application of a conditioned stimulus, in which the excitation of the center perceiving the conditioned stimulus, spreads through a temporary connection to the center perceiving the unconditioned stimulus and a response occurs through efferent pathways (e.g., saliva secretion to the action of a light stimulus); 2) according to P.K. Anokhin.

The diagram shows the mechanism of conditioned reflex emergence according to the convergent theory of P.K. Anokhin. The simultaneous action of conditioned (P1) and unconditioned (P2) stimuli (reinforcement) excites subcortical centers (P1 and P2), resulting in the involvement of the reticular formation (RF). From the RF there are two streams of impulses (convergence occurs) to the cortex of the large hemispheres, where excitation occurs simultaneously all the way from the center perceiving the conditioned stimulus (K1) to the center perceiving the unconditioned stimulus (K2). With repeated reinforcement in the cortex of the large hemispheres there is a temporary connection between K1 and K2, due to which there is a reaction to the action of an isolated conditioned stimulus. With repeated reinforcement, a temporal connection between the two centers occurs.

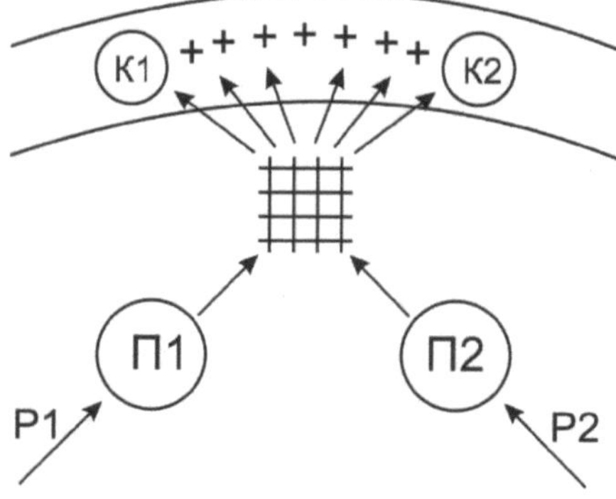

Lecture 36.

Topic: Inhibition in GND: types and mechanism of their occurrence. Sleep and dreams. Physiological basis of hypnotic states.

Objective - to know the physiological basis and features of different types of inhibition of GND and its adaptive role.

The objectives are.

(a) Give the basic theories of sleep;

b) to show the interaction of the PMA, hypothalamic parts of the brain and the RF in the mechanisms of sleep and wakefulness (P.K. Anokhin);

c) reveal the physiological phases and types of sleep; show the physiological basis of dreams and hypnotic states.

Content:

Inhibition of higher nervous activity - there are two types of inhibition of GND: 1) unconditional, or external and 2) conditional, or internal. Unconditional inhibition is directed to the neurons forming the center of a given reflex. Conditional inhibition is directed to the temporal connection in the cortex of the large hemispheres. The following types of unconditional inhibition are distinguished: 1) external inhibition - arises as a result of an additional external stimulus: a) extinguishing external inhibition, when an additional stimulus produces an orienting reflex, causing inhibition of conditioned reflex activity of the cortex of the large hemispheres. With repeated application of this stimulus, the inhibitory reaction fades away; b) permanent external inhibition, when an additional stimulus causes a damaging effect (pain) and inhibition of conditioned reflex activity of the cortex of the large hemispheres occurs; 2) limit inhibition (guarding according to I.P. Pavlov) - occurs under the action of a prolonged stimulus or under the action of superstrong stimuli and has a guarding character. For external inhibition to occur, an additional stimulus is required, and the inhibition is prohibitive when the same stimulus that causes conditioned reflex activity is applied.

For conditional inhibition it is necessary to first develop a conditioned reflex (a temporary connection in the cortex of the large hemispheres). The main condition for the emergence of conditioned inhibition is the cessation of reinforcement of the conditioned signal by the action of the unconditioned signal. Depending on how the reinforcement is terminated, the following types of conditioned inhibition are distinguished:

1) extinction inhibition - occurs at complete cessation of reinforcement of the conditioned signal by the action of the unconditional stimulus, after a long isolated application of the conditioned signal (without reinforcement) the reflex disappears.

2) delayed inhibition - occurs due to delayed reinforcement. After the development of a conditioned reflex, we continue to periodically reinforce the conditioned signal with the action of the unconditioned signal, but with a delay, so when the conditioned signal is applied in isolation, the reflex does not appear immediately, but with some delay.

3) conditioned brake - after the development of a conditioned reflex, we add another stimulus (indifferent) to the conditioned signal without reinforcement in this combination. Very soon there will be a reflex to the isolated application of the conditioned signal, but in combination with another stimulus there is no reaction. This other stimulus is a conditioned brake for the main conditioned signal and the conditioned reflex stops;

4) differentiation inhibition ensures the distinction of signals that are close in nature, one of which is reinforced by the action of an unconditioned stimulus, and the other is not. With repeated reinforcement

we develop a conditioned reflex to the sound 10000 Hz. After the development of a conditioned reflex, the reaction occurs to the action of the sound of 8000 Hz. In the future, we will periodically reinforce the action of the 10000 Hz sound with the action of the unconditioned stimulus, and we will not reinforce the action of the 8000 Hz sound. As a result, the reaction only to 10000 Hz (D) is preserved, and the reaction to the sound of 8000 Hz disappears, i.e. differentiation inhibition occurs.

Sleep is one of the varieties of inhibition of GND. Sleep is a periodic physiological process characterized by the shutdown of consciousness and a significant weakening of the body's connection with the external environment. Sleep is a spilt inhibition of the cerebral cortex and subcortical structures of the brain with preservation of excitation in vital centers. Sleep is a special form of activity of the cortex of the large hemispheres when no signals from analyzers are received. When recording the electroencephalogram during sleep, it was found that during sleep all four waves can be reflected, differing in frequency and amplitude (amplitude decreases with increasing frequency): 1) alpha rhythm (frequency 8-13 Hz, amplitude about 50µV), found in healthy people with closed eyes in the awake state; 2) beta rhythm (frequency 14-40 Hz, amplitude up to 15µV), found in healthy people with open eyes in the awake state; 3) theta rhythm (frequency 4-6 Hz, amplitude 100µV); delta rhythm (frequency 0.5-3 Hz, amplitude more than 100µV). Theta and delta rhythms are found in deep anesthesia, cerebral hypoxia, and deep sleep. Conventionally, EEG rhythms can be divided into fast (alpha and beta) rhythms that occur in the awake state and slow (theta and delta) rhythms that occur in deep sleep.

Thus, two types of sleep are distinguished according to the waves on the EEG: 1) slow-wave type of sleep, where the theta and delta rhythms (slow waves) are predominantly noted on the EEG. This type of sleep is characterized by a decrease in respiratory rate, heart rate, muscle tone, ATP formation and anabolic processes predominate, STG, melatonin, paratgormone and ADH secretion is enhanced. In this type of sleep there are dreams of a logical nature, are associated with the activity of the left hemisphere, there is dreaming, dreaming, nightmares and night terrors, teeth grinding; 2) REM sleep (paradoxical sleep, sleep accompanied by rapid eye movements - BDG-sleep) - is characterized by a paradoxical state of the body: compared to rest in the waking state, some functions in this type of sleep are activated, others are inhibited. This type of sleep is characterized by a "vegetative storm" (increase in HR, BP, respiratory rate, blood flow of the pelvic organs and genitals) and rapid eyeball movement, fast waves (alpha and beta) appear on the EEG. In this type of sleep 80% of people have vivid, imaginative, emotional dreams associated with the activation of the right hemisphere; information is transferred into long-term memory. In this type of sleep, there is a maximum drop in the tone of skeletal muscles of the limbs and trunk, a decrease in body temperature, STH and melatonin secretion, sharply reduced secretory and peristaltic activity of the digestive tract.

According to I.M. Sechenov, dreams are unprecedented combinations of former impressions. From this definition follows: 1) one can see in a dream what one has seen in the waking state (old impressions); 2) a blind person from birth "sees" in a dream only sounds, and a deaf-mute from birth sees visual images without sound accompaniment. Each person sees 4-5 dreams during sleep - this is related to the amount of rapid-onset type of sleep. Memorization of dreams occurs when a person wakes up after a REM sleep type. People who wake up during slow-wave type of sleep claim that they either don't dream at all or see dreams very rarely. During dreaming, cerebral blood flow increases, the frequency of impulse discharges of the brainstem, cerebral cortex and thalamus increases.

Dreams are accompanied by rapid eye movements and pronounced changes in autonomic indices. The origin of dreams can be explained by the activation of traces of long-term memory associated even with random impressions of long ago, while the impressions of the previous day have little influence on the content of dreams.

Hypnosis is from the Greek meaning sleep. The scientific era of hypnosis is associated with the name of English surgeon D. Breda, who said that hypnosis is nothing but a nervous sleep. According to I.P. Pavlov - it is a partial sleep, in this case in the cortex of the large hemispheres retains a focus of excitation formed by the hypnotizer and through this focus of excitation hypnotizer can affect the function of any subcortical formation. This focus of excitation I.P. Pavlov called the watchdog center, or report zone. In humans, three stages of hypnosis are distinguished: superficial, middle and deep (somnambulism stage). Hypnosis is widely used in medicine to treat diseases associated with functional disorders, can be used as an anesthetic agent, as well as for the treatment of all sorts of hysterical syndromes (hysterical paralysis, hysterical blindness, etc.). Complex dynamic relationships in hypnosis are formed between the conscious and unconscious spheres.

Lecture 37.

Topic: Emotions, their importance for the body, classification, theories of emergence.

Objective - to know the physiological basis and characteristics of emotions.

The objectives are.

(a) Uncover the autonomic and somatic components of emotion;

b) give a classification of emotions;

c) show the participation of central structures in the formation of emotions;

Content:

Emotion is from Latin *emoveo, emovere - to excite, excite. Emotions* are subjective reactions to external and internal stimuli, including the results of one's own activity, accompanied by expressed subjective experiences. Emotions are special mental functions of a person. Emotion is a relation of actual need to the probability of satisfaction of this need: with increasing probability of satisfaction of this actual need there are positive emotions, and with decreasing probability of satisfaction of the actual need there are negative emotions. The biological significance of emotions is that they perform a signaling and regulatory function. The signaling function consists in that they signal about usefulness or harmfulness of the given influence on an organism, and also success or not success of the performed action. Regulatory function of emotion consists in the fact that it forms the activity to stop or strengthen the action of stimuli.

Theories of emotions - I. Peripheral theory (W. James, C. Lange) according to this theory emotions are due to awareness in the activity of visceral and somatic systems. "We cry not because we are sad, but we are sad because we cry". According to this theory it is primary that we cry and realization that we cry promotes occurrence of emotion of sadness, that is primary are changes in peripheral organs and realization of these changes causes occurrence of emotions. II. Central theories consider emotions as a result of activation of brain structures: a) thalamic - excitation, coming into the thalamus, is divided into two streams - one goes to the cortex and causes subjective experiences (emotions), and the second goes to the hypothalamus and causes physiological reactions (W. Kennon, V.M. Bekhterev); b) hypothalamic - pleasure and punishment centers (W. Hess, D. Olds); c) limbic system (hippocampus, mamillary bodies, anterior thalamic nuclei, cingulate gyrus). Currently, the role of various brain structures in the formation of emotions can be systematized as follows: 1) hypothalamus is the main structure forming the actual need of the organism and emotions: lateral nuclei form positive emotions, and medial nuclei form negative emotions; 2) amygdaloid body of temporal lobe provides allocation of dominant motivation. Electrical stimulation of the amygdala is accompanied by the emergence of the emotion of fear, anger, rage. Removal of the amygdala suppresses aggressiveness; 3) hippocampus - here the memory of experienced emotions is formed; 4) frontal cortex is involved in the formation of higher emotions related to social relations and creativity; 5) temporal cortex is involved in recognizing emotional reactions of other people; 6) cingulate gyrus has the most extensive connections with other parts of the brain, is involved in the coordination of other brain systems involved in the formation of emotions; 7) limbic system: (a) Most of the above structures are part of Peipetz's limbic circle (from the hippocampus through the vault to the mamillary bodies, from them to the anterior nuclei of the thalamus, from it to the cingulate gyrus and from it through the parahippocampal gyrus back to the hippocampus). This circle plays a major role in the formation of emotions, learning and memory; b) the other limbic circle (from the amygdala to the mamillary bodies of the hypothalamus, from them to the limbic area of the midbrain and back to the amygdala) is involved in the formation of emotions accompanying aggressive-defensive, food and sexual reactions; 8) the role of the left and right hemispheres: a) the left hemisphere controls positive emotions, responds faster to slides expressing joy, reduces the degree of anxiety; b) the right hemisphere causes a shift towards negative emotions, responds faster to slides expressing sadness, recognizes emotional intonation of speech and voice coloration. The role of various neurotransmitters in emotion formation should also be noted: 1) stimulation of adrenergic (blue spot), dopaminergic (black matter) and serotoninergic (central gray matter) brain systems (increase in the content of norepinephrine, serotonin and dopamine) is accompanied by the formation of positive emotions; 2) decrease in the level of noradrenaline and dopamine leads to feelings of longing, anxiety and fear; 3) acetylcholine is a trigger mediator of aggressive behavior, and serotonin inhibits aggression; 4) endorphins and enkephalins exert their influence through opiate receptors and participate in the formation of positive emotions during orientation and exploration reactions. III. Biological theory (P.K. Anokhin, 1948), which considers emotions from the standpoint of functional systems of the organism and as if unites all theories (p.81, Fig.Zh5). The trigger mechanism according to this theory is the deviation of some final useful adaptive result (KPPP) from the optimal level, which forms an actual need of the organism, which can be satisfied by the functional reserves of the organism by changing the function of the corresponding effectors (in this case there is no emotion). If this need is not satisfied by changing the work of all effectors responsible for the given CPPP, then the brain structures belonging to the Peipets circle are involved in the process, which leads to the emergence of a negative emotion and the cortex of the large hemispheres is involved in the process (due to impulses from the cingulate gyrus), and purposeful behavior occurs. In case of adequate behavior, the actual need of the organism is satisfied (CPPP returns to the optimal level) and the negative emotion is replaced by a positive one. IV. Need-information theory (P.V. Simonov, 1984) - according to this theory, in order to satisfy any actual need of the organism, certain information (necessary information - IN) is required. In this case, the organism has existing information (includes knowledge, skills, energy resources, time, which the organism has to satisfy its need - IS). Positive emotions arise if the probability of achieving the goal increases, when IS is greater than IN. Negative emotions arise when the probability of achieving the goal decreases, when IS is greater than IS.

Autonomic shifts in emotions. It is established that in fear we become pale, pupils dilate, sweat appears, mouth dries up. In joy, the face turns red. In 1878 for the first time was discovered effect: if a cat tied to the machine to show a dog, then in the urine it detects sugar. W. Kenon in 1923 gave a response to this phenomenon by activation of the sympathetic section of the ANS. Sympathetic nervous system provides the activity of the organism aimed at urgent adaptation to changed conditions, it as if prepares the body for defense, attack, work.

The parasympathetic system provides the functions necessary to restore the disturbed balance in the body, to restore its strength and resources.

The universality of emotions is that they are able to unite all functional systems capable of providing a holistic reaction of the organism to this or that impact.

P.V. Simonov - emotion is a special mechanism to compensate for the lack, deficiency of information necessary for the organism to organize actions to meet a particular need. Thus fear is an emotion arising from the lack of information necessary to ensure successful defense against the enemy. Rage - lack of information to organize a successful fight. Fright - lack of information about the source and size of an unexpected threat. Positive emotions according to Simonov arise when the brain receives excessive information compared to the expected. Since the hypothalamus is actively involved in the formation of emotion, so any emotion is accompanied by an autonomic component. Closely related to the function of the sympathetic nervous system is the function of the cerebral layer of the adrenal glands, released adrenaline and noradrenaline - increased heart rate, release of sugar from the depot (hyperglycemia). Related to the function of the parasympathetic nervous system is the function of the pancreas, releasing insulin, which binds glucose and transfers it to the depot. Thus, during emotion there is activation of two systems in the body: 1) sympathoadrenal and 2) vagoinsulin. It has been found that in different animals during emotions there are predominantly either sympathetic (in dogs, cats) or parasympathetic (in rabbits) effects. The nature of the emotion can determine the type of autonomic response: in fear and anger, sympathetic reactions prevail, and in pleasant emotions, parasympathetic reactions prevail (in fear, we turn pale, and in praise, we blush). During emotions both systems are activated, but one of them prevails. Observation of British scientists during the war in bomb shelters showed that some people in fear pale, others - blush. It turned out that the same emotion can give different vegetative effect depending on what subsequent action it is associated with. If the emotion of fear ends in flight, the sympathetic system predominates. If fear is associated with freezing in place - parasympathetic shifts. Thus vegetative shifts are formed not only on the basis of emotional experience, but also in connection with the future need of the organism in this or that behavior.

It was found out that in different emotions there are different ratios of adrenaline and noradrenaline release. In animals in the state of fear and anxiety - adrenaline production prevails; in aggressive behavior - noradrenaline. Endocrine and vegetative shifts during emotions form the basis of emotional stress.

<h1 style="text-align:center">Lecture 38.</h1>

<h2 style="text-align:center"><u>Topic: Biological motivations, theories of their origin. Drug addiction as one of the types of pathological motivation, mechanisms. Importance of start and stop zones, opiate receptors</u></h2>

Objective - to know the physiological bases of biological motivations, the leading role of internal needs in the formation of biological motivations. To know the physiological bases underlying the emergence of drug addiction.

The objectives are.

(a) Review existing theories of the emergence of biological motivations;

b) indicate the role of internal needs in the formation of biological motivations.

(c) Identify the role of internal needs in the formation of drug abuse;

d) give the importance of start and stop zones, opiate receptors in the formation of drug addiction.

Content:

When some internal need arises, a motivational arousal occurs, which leads to the formation of ARD. After that, the body systems that should lead to the satisfaction of this need begin to be activated. The exhaustion of internal reserves leads to purposeful behavior of animals in the environment. This search stops in the case of adequate reinforcement, i.e., when the parameters of reinforcement coincide with the parameters of the ARD model that emerged on the basis of motivational arousal. The result of this coincidence is positive emotions.

Any internal need is specific and so the search is directed toward special stimuli that satisfy that internal need. Very characteristic in this respect is the example of Wilkins and Richter (1940): they observed a boy with a congenital tumor of the adrenal glands - his body as a result was not able to retain sodium ions From birth, this child had been anxious and would not calm down after eating regular food. Later he began to prefer salty food and quickly learned to ask for salt with the help of gestures. It is characteristic that the first word pronounced to him was "salt". Salted food and everything connected with salt became for this child the main goal of his short life.

In this respect, the experience developed in the laboratory of P.K. Anokhin is indicative. Four groups of rats were taken: 1) these rats were deprived of food for 1-2 days; 2) - were deprived of water for the same period; 3) were fed with salty food during this period; 4) adrenal glands were removed from these rats. After this preparation, the animals are let into the cage where they are offered a choice of food, water and salt. After some time, the animals take their place accordingly to their dominant motivation, i.e., where they have the opportunity to satisfy their initial need: 1g. - at the feeder with food; 2 gr. - at water; 3 gr. - at fresh water; 4 gr. - at salt.

Thus the initial internal need absolutely determines the behavior of each animal in the external environment.

American physiologists Aldzi, Braley and Lilly implanted microelectrodes in various areas of the brain and discovered, thanks to experiments on self-irritation, that there are neurons that animals constantly seek to irritate. These neurons were called start zones. They also discovered neurons that animals avoid irritating - stop zones. The reactions arising from irritation of these zones can be represented in the form of the following scheme:

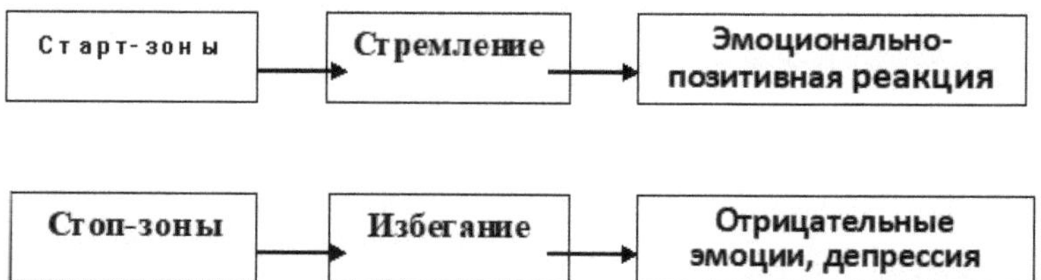

Researchers Wicks, Thomson and Denau conducted experiments on rats and monkeys to train them to reactions of varying complexity. They found that the learning process was much faster if the reinforcement was given with an intravenous infusion of narcotic drugs.

In 1975, Scottish researchers Kosterlitz and Hughes discovered opioid peptides (endorphins and enkephalins - drugs produced in our bodies) in brain extracts that block opiate receptors and cause hedonic effects.

Based on the above, it is possible to visualize the processes that occur in the body when using an external drug in the form of the following scheme:

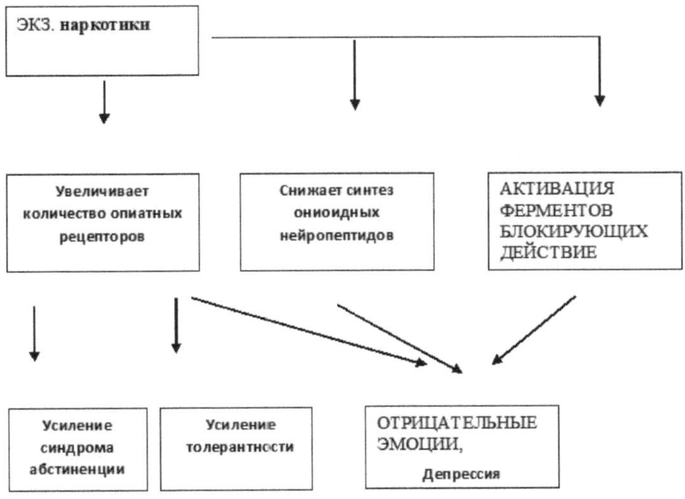

This scheme shows that when using a drug, the number of opiate receptors increases in direct connection, which leads on the one hand to increased tolerance (to get hedonic effect it is necessary to increase the dose every time), and on the other hand to increased withdrawal syndrome (i.e. the previous dose does not satisfy). According to feedback, the synthesis of opioid neuropeptides is sharply reduced, because the dose of external drug is 100 times higher than the dose of internal drug synthesized in the body. On the other hand, there is activation of enzymes that block the effect of the drug (due to the large dose). Thus, an increase in the number of opiate receptors, a decrease in the synthesis of opioid neuropeptides and the activation of enzymes that block the action of the drug leads to negative emotions (depression), which disappear only when the actual need is satisfied, i.e. the use of a drug - a vicious circle.

The emergence of pathological motivation in drug use (drug addiction) can be explained with the help of the body's functional systems (FUS). Among all FUS, the dominant one is the FUS that maintains optimal drug content in the body (endorphins and enkephalins). The fact is that the metabolism of hypothalamic neurons is closely related to a certain concentration of opioid neuropeptides (the final beneficial adaptive outcome - KPPP). The hypothalamus is the peutzmecker of all biological motivations and before any behavior can be performed to satisfy an actual need of the organism (return of KPPR to the optimal level), an optimal concentration of opioid neuropeptides must be created. When drugs from outside the body are used, the synthesis of opioid neuropeptides is inhibited by feedback (the external drug dose is almost a hundred times higher than the concentration of neuropeptides). With frequent drug use, the function of neurons producing opioid neuropeptides atrophies. The person is forced to use drugs from the outside.

PATHOLOGICAL STAGING

1. Stimulation of positive-emotional response (addictive, addictive);
2. Mental dependence (withdrawal, tolerance);
3. Physical dependence (impaired production of liberins and statins, changes in the tone of the ANS).

Lecture 39.

Topic: Adaptation of the organism to various factors, mechanisms and phases. Stress and its stages. Classification of stress and stressors. General adaptation syndrome and its mechanism. Stress - realizing and stress - limiting systems.

Objective - to know the concept of adaptation, its mechanisms and phases.

The objectives are.

(a) Show the mechanisms of adaptation of the organism to various factors;

b) specify the phases cf adaptation (equilibrating, transitional and stable) and the processes occurring in each phase;

c) reveal the general acaptation syndrome and its mechanism;

d) give a classification of stressors and stressors;

e) specify stress-realizing and stress-limiting systems.

Content:

Adaptation is the adaptation of the organism to changes in natural, industrial and domestic conditions. The purpose of adaptation is to restore homeostasis (relative dynamic constancy of the internal environment and physiological functions) of the organism under changed environmental conditions. Adaptation capabilities of the organism are a measure of its health. There are three phases of adaptation: 1f - "emergency phase" - develops at the very beginning. In this phase there is a mobilization of systems reacting to the change of environmental conditions due to the activation of the sympathoadrenal system (the tone of the sympathetic section of the autonomous nervous system and the function of the brain layer of the adrenal glands increases. The level of mobilization of systems can exceed the level of functional reserve and then there can be a "crash", i.e. a violation in this system. 2f - transitional phase of adaptation. In this phase, the search for the body systems to the optimal level of functioning, corresponding to the changed conditions. At the same time, the intensity of hormonal shifts decreases, the function of a number of systems initially involved in the reaction gradually decreases. 3f - steady (stable) phase of adaptation, or resistance, as in this phase increases the resistance of the organism to the action of factors caused by changes in environmental conditions. In this phase, a new level of activity of tissue cell membrane elements is noted, which are reorganized due to the temporary activation of auxiliary systems in the first phase of adaptation. At the same time, auxiliary systems can function at the initial level (before the change of habitat conditions) or at a level lower than the initial one.

General adaptation syndrome - in 1936 G. Sellier formulated his idea of stress and introduced a new concept "Syndrome caused by different damaging agents", or "general adaptation syndrome", or "biological stress syndrome" - it is a nonspecific neurohumoral reaction of the organism to the action of stressors (all factors of external and internal environment that are dangerous to the health and integrity of the organism). The general adaptation syndrome, or stress is usually called the reaction of activation of homeostatic mechanisms, and the processes that ensure the adaptation of the organism to activity in new conditions is called adaptation. The organism responds to any extreme stimulus (stressor) with a complex reaction. This reaction consists of specific (adequate to this stimulus) and general nonspecific (characteristic of any stressor). The general nonspecific reaction arising under any stressor is a physiological manifestation of the general adaptation syndrome.

Stress - from the English word stress - tension. Currently, there are several definitions of stress: 1) stress is a nonspecific reaction of the organism to any external demand (G. Sellier, 1974); 2) stress is a reaction of the organism to a significant stimulus; 3) stress is a way to achieve restiveness (stability) of the organism when it is exposed to a damaging factor. A distinction is made between physical stress and emotional (psychogenic) stress. In physical stress there is a defense against the effects of physical factors (hypoxia, heat, cold, burn, trauma, etc.). In emotional stress there is a defense against psychogenic factors that cause negative emotions. G. Sellier introduced the concept of eustress and distress. Eustress (literally good stress) is characterized by the fact that the protective reaction of the organism proceeds without damage to it, painlessly. Distress (excessive stress) is characterized by the fact that the protection of the organism occurs with damage to it, with weakening of its capabilities. Stages of stress: 1st. - the stage of anxiety is divided into two phases: a) phase of shock - short-lived follows immediately after the action of the stimulus. It is characterized by CNS inhibition, decrease in BP, muscle tone, body temperature, glucose level, leukocytes. The resistance of the body is reduced. If the force of the stimulus is great, death may occur in this phase. If the force of stress is small, the phase of shock is absent and immediately comes the phase of counter-shock, during which the resistance of the organism increases; 2st. - the stage of resistance is characterized by maximum resistance of the organism to the stressor. In this stage the tension of regulatory systems decreases; Stage 3 - the stage of exhaustion occurs under the action of strong and long stressors. At this stage resistance of the organism decreases, adaptation diseases occur.

Stressors are all factors in the external and internal environment that cause a stress response that are dangerous to the health and integrity of the body. Such factors include: 1) harmful environmental stimuli (gassiness, radiation, heat, hypoxia, etc.); 2) disruption of physiological processes in the body (all diseases); 3) working under time pressure; 4) working under conditions of risk to one's own life or others; 5) perceived threat to life; 6) isolation and confinement; 7) ostracism (exile, persecution), group pressure; 8) lack of control over events; 9) lack of purpose in life; 10) deprivation - lack of stimuli. Sellier believed that lack of purpose is one of the strongest stressors causing the development of pathological process (gastric ulcer, myocardial infarction, hypertension).

Stress-implementing system is a regulatory complex that activates and coordinates all changes in the organism that constitute the adaptive response to stressors.   Stress-realizing systems include: 1) activation of the sympathetic section of the autonomic nervous system (due to activation of the posterior nuclei of the hypothalamus), which leads to an increase in the function of the SSS, respiration and skeletal muscles. This system due to limited mediator reserves acts for a short period of time. At longer action of stressor the following system is switched on; 2) adrenal medulla - release of adrenaline and noradrenaline into blood, as a result of which blood pressure increases, cardiac output increases, blood flow in idle muscles and organs decreases, level of free fatty acids, triglycerides, cholesterol, glucose increases. Often these two systems are combined as the sympatho-adrenal system.   If the stressor continues to act, other endocrine mechanisms (endocrine axes) are activated; 3) the adrenocortical system is the central link of the stress-realizing system. This mechanism is activated if the sympatho-adrenal system is ineffective: cortex - hypothalamus - release of corticoliberin - anterior lobe of the pituitary gland - release of ACTH - adrenal cortex - release of glucocorticoids (cortisol, hydrocortisone). These hormones significantly increase the energy reserve: the level of glucose and free fatty acids increases. With increased ACTH release, aldosterone production increases, which increases reabsorption of sodium ions, resulting in increased water reabsorption and increased blood pressure; 4) simultaneously with the activation of the adrenocortical system there is activation of the somatotropic system: cortex - hypothalamus - release of somatoliberin - anterior lobe of pituitary - release of somatotropic hormone - liver formation of somatomedins - increases resistance to insulin, accelerates mobilization of stored fats in the body, which ultimately leads to an increase in blood glucose and free fatty acids; 5) activation of the thyroid system may occur: cortex - hypothalamus - release of thyreoliberin - anterior lobe of the pituitary gland - release of thyroid hormone - thyroid gland - release of thyroid hormones of the thyroid gland (triiodothyronine and thyroxine), which increase tissue sensitivity to catecholamines, increase the level of energy formation, activate the activity of the heart, there is an increase in blood pressure; 6) activation of the parasympathetic system is not sufficiently studied: It is known that this system is involved in hyperinsulinemia.

Stresslimiting system - in the process of evolution in the organism there appeared mechanisms preventing the emergence of side effects of stressors or reducing the intensity of their impact on the body, preventing the development of damage, including psychosomatic diseases. The work of these systems is carried out by the mechanism of self-regulation and negative feedback. Stress-limiting systems include: 1) melatonin, an epiphysis hormone, coordinates the interaction of the nervous, endocrine and immune systems in response to stress. This hormone inhibits the production of corticoliberin in the hypothalamus, ACTH in the pituitary gland, and steroidogenesis in the adrenal glands when glucocorticoid secretion is very high. Melatonin stimulates activation of other stress-limiting systems, is a powerful endogenous antioxidant, inhibits lipid peroxidation and protects proteins and genetic apparatus of the cell from free radical damage; 2) GABAergic system - has its effect on CNS and peripheral nerve endings, limits secretion of corticoliberin, ACTH and release of norepinephrine and adrenaline. This system prevents the triggering of the stress response; 3) the opioidergic system, which includes opioid peptides (endorphins, enkephalins, dinorphins) released from central neurons of the CNS, adenohypophysis and adrenal medulla. This system limits the damaging effects of catecholamines and inhibits the production of corticoliberin, vasopressin, oxytacin, glucocorticoids, and catecholamines. In addition, being a component of the antinociceptive system reduce pain sensitivity and anxiety and thereby reduces the intensity of the emotional reaction that triggers the stress response; 4) nitric oxide - released simultaneously with noradrenaline from the endings of sympathetic neurons and prevents vasospasm, increases the activity of antioxidant enzymes and increases the synthesis of heat shock proteins (stress proteins) that prevent denaturation of cell proteins; 5) local tissue stress-limiting systems are represented by substances formed in the tissues themselves: prostaglandins, adenosine, antioxidants (proteins - ceruloplasmin, myoglobin, transferrin; enzymes - superoxide dismutase, catalase, glutathione peroxidase; small molecules - glutathione, vitamins C, E, betacarotins). Glucocorticoids, which are released under the action of stress, contribute to the activation of lipid peroxidation with the formation of free radicals, which lead to the activation of many biochemical reactions in the cell, which disrupts its vital activity. Antioxidants are endogenous "quenchers" of these free radical processes; 6) parasympathetic system - its activation under stress is the most important mechanism of protection against side effects of glucocorticoids and other participants of stress reaction: cortex - hypothalamus - parasympathetic centers of brainstem and sacral spinal cord. In addition to natural triggering of this mechanism, it is possible to artificially increase the activity of this system, which can be used as a preventive measure in the fight against excessive effects of stress: moderate physical activity (after it the tone of the parasympathetic system increases), muscle relaxation, meditation, change of breathing (transition to diaphragmatic breathing increases the activity of the parasympathetic part of the autonomic nervous system).

Lecture 40.

Topic: Mental and physical performance of a person, ways of its determination.

Objective - to know the concept of physical and mental performance and how to determine them.

The objectives are.

(a) Show the phases of physical performance;

b) familiarize with the methods of determining physical and mental performance.

Content:

Work capacity is one of the basic concepts of work physiology. Workability is a person's potential ability to perform physical (physical work capacity - WP) or mental (mental work capacity - MW) work for a certain period of time. Workability depends on many factors, including mental and physical development, the degree of training, the degree of adaptation to physical and mental labor, all factors of working conditions, and health status.

PHYSICAL PERFORMANCE

There are the following methods for assessing FRs:

a. Determination of FR by means of Cooper's test - in this case, the examinee must run a distance of 2400 meters for a time.

b. PWC170 test - determine the load at which the heart rate reaches 170 beats/min. This is considered the optimal load, because up to 170 beats/min the relationship between the power of the load and heart rate is direct, and after 170 beats/min this relationship is broken. The PWC170 test is carried out in two ways: a) a load is given on a bicycle ergometer and every 2 minutes we increase the power of the load (at the end of the second minute we

172

measure the pulse rate) until the pulse reaches 170 ud/min; b) according to V.L. Karpman - at first we give one load, which the researcher performs for 5 minutes, then rest for 3 minutes and the second load is given, which is also performed for 5 minutes. We record the power of both loads, the pulse rate at the first and second loads (in 4mi 30 sec after the beginning of the load) and by a special formula we calculate the load at which the pulse will reach 179 beats/min.

c.   To determine the maximum oxygen consumption (MOC). We determine the oxygen consumption at loads of different power until the increase in load does not lead to an increase in oxygen consumption. Up to a certain load capacity, the MPC varies in direct proportion - as the load capacity increases, the oxygen consumption increases.

d.   Step test - a 50 cm high step is used. The test subject performs two loads with different frequency of climbing the step and descending. The loads are performed for 5 min each. Between loads rest 3 min. We record HR (pulse rate) after each load, then according to a special formula we calculate the physical activity of the test subject.

e.   FR can be assessed by characterizing the functional reserve of the organism, which can be determined by correlation rhythmograms or variation variation of cardiointervals at rest and at loads of different power.

MENTAL PERFORMANCE

Mental performance can be defined as follows:

1. The study of memory - short-term and long-term. The greater the memory capacity, the greater the mental efficiency of a person.

2. Attention research - a direct correlation between attention and mental performance. Attention can be assessed by the following tests: a) a proofreading test; b) using broken lines; c) a red-black table of different levels of complexity: Krepelin test

3. The study of logical ability is determined by; a) ciphering; b) identifying a pattern; c) identifying analogies

The effectiveness of any work capacity is limited by fatigue. Fatigue is a decrease in performance caused by previous work, which has a temporary character. If it occurs during SD, we speak of mental fatigue, and if it occurs during FR, we speak of physical fatigue. The state of fatigue is manifested in the change of physiological processes, in the decrease of labor productivity, in the change of mental status. These changes are determined by dynamic registration of various vegetative indices, as well as by the study of mental status using various psycho-physiological tests.

List of literature used

1. Khalimova F.T. Short course on normal physiology Chisinau: LAP LAMBERT, 2023, 221 p. ISBN 978-620-5-63127-0.

2. Atlas of normal physiology\ Edited by N.A. Agajanian. - M. Higher School, 1987. - 351c.

3. Normal physiology. Course of physiology of functional systems \ Under the editorship of K.V. Sudakov. - M. MIA, 1999. - 718c.

4. Normal physiology. Textbook, ed. by V.A. Polyantsev. - M. Medicine, 1989. - 239c.

5. Fundamentals of human physiology. Textbook / N.A. Agajanian. M - RUDN.- 468 p.

6. Fundamentals of human physiology. Textbook in 3 volumes \ Edited by Acad.   RAMS B.I. B.T. Tkachenko. SPb., 1994. - Vol. 1 - 567c, St. Petersburg, 1994, - Vol. 2 - 413c. - M. Litera, 1998, Vol.3 - 474c

7. Features of physiology of children. Textbook, ed. by V.M. Smirnov. - M. RGMU, 1993. - 168c

8. Human Physiology. Compendium \ Edited by Acad. RAMS B.I. Tkachenko, Prof. V.F. Pyatin, Samara. House of Press, 2003. - 496c.

9. Physiology. Fundamentals and functional systems. Course of lectures \ Edited by K.V. Sudakov. - I. Medicine, 1999. - 784c.

10. Shukurov F.A., Halimova F.T. Course of lectures on normal physiology, volume one. Chisinau: LAP LAMBERT, 2023, 237 p. ISBN 978-620-5-63277-2.

11. Shukurov F.A., Halimova F.T. Normal physiology: Textbook for students of medical universities Mauritius: LAP LAMBERT, 2020. - 345 c. - ISBN 978-620-2-80134-8. - EDN RVIRER.

12. Shukurov F.A., Halimova F.T. Physiology in schemes and drawings. Chisinau: LAP LAMBERT, 2022, 158 p. ISBN 978-620-5-51354-5.

13. Orlov R.S., Nozdrachev A.D. Normal physiology. Textbook for universities, publishing group "GEOTAR-Media", Moscow, 2005, 687 pp.

14. Shukurov F.A. Physiology of Man. Dushanbe, 2009, 320 p

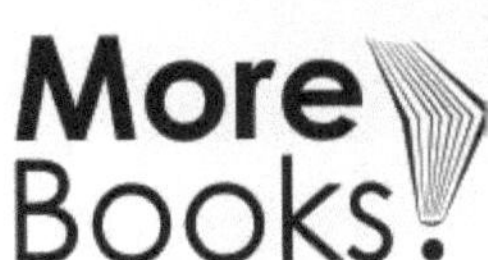

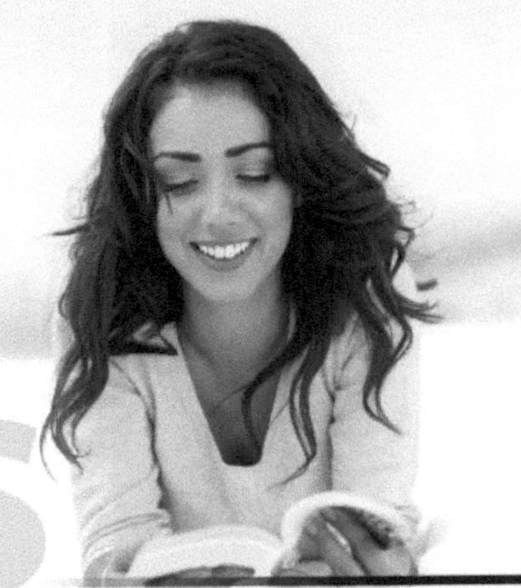

I want morebooks!

Buy your books fast and straightforward online - at one of world's fastest growing online book stores! Environmentally sound due to Print-on-Demand technologies.

Buy your books online at
www.morebooks.shop

Kaufen Sie Ihre Bücher schnell und unkompliziert online – auf einer der am schnellsten wachsenden Buchhandelsplattformen weltweit! Dank Print-On-Demand umwelt- und ressourcenschonend produziert.

Bücher schneller online kaufen
www.morebooks.shop

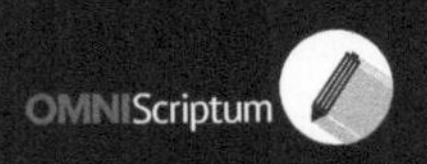

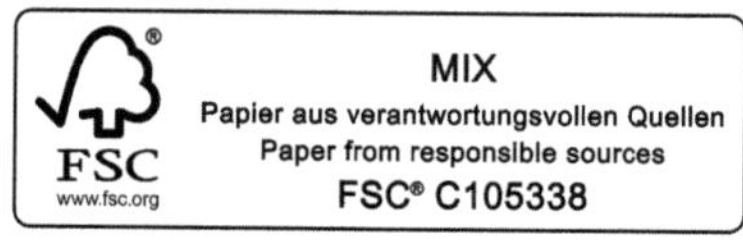

Printed by Books on Demand GmbH, Norderstedt / Germany